Respiratory Care Pearls

Respiratory Care Pearls

FRANK A. MAZZAGATTI, M.S.A., R.R.T.
Associate Technical Director
Respiratory Therapy Department
The Brookdale University Hospital and Medical Center
Brooklyn, New York
Adjunct Instructor in Cardiorespiratory Sciences
Allied Health Sciences Department
Molloy College
Rockville Centre, New York

LEON C. LEBOWITZ, B.A., R.R.T.
Technical Director
Respiratory Therapy Department
The Brookdale University Hospital and Medical Center
Brooklyn, New York

NEIL W. SCHLUGER, M.D.
Assistant Professor of Medicine
New York University School of Medicine
Director, Bellevue Hospital Chest Clinic
New York, New York

Series Editors

STEVEN A. SAHN, M.D.
Professor of Medicine and Director
Division of Pulmonary and
  Critical Care Medicine
Medical University of South Carolina
Charleston, South Carolina

JOHN E. HEFFNER, M.D.
Professor of Clinical Medicine
University of Arizona Health Sciences Center
Chairman, Academic Internal Medicine
St. Joseph's Hospital and Medical Center
Phoenix, Arizona

HANLEY & BELFUS, INC./Philadelphia

Publisher: HANLEY & BELFUS, INC.
            Medical Publishers
            210 S. 13th Street
            Philadelphia, PA 19107
            (215) 546-7293
            (800) 962-1892
            FAX (215) 790-9330

United States sales and distribution:

            MOSBY
            11830 Westline Industrial Drive
            St. Louis, MO 63146

Library of Congress Cataloging-in-Publication Data

Mazzagatti, Frank, 1966-
    Respiratory Care Pearls / Frank Mazzagatti, Leon Lebowitz, Neil Schluger.
        p.   cm. – (The Pearls Series®)
    Includes bibliographical references and index.
    ISBN 1-56053-204-1 (alk. paper)
    1. Respiratory organs—Diseases—Case studies. 2. Respiratory therapy—
Case studies. I. Lebowitz, Leon, 1949-   II. Schluger, Neil W., 1959-
III. Title. IV. Series.
    [DNLM: 1. Lung Diseases—therapy—problems. 2. Lung Diseases—therapy—
case studies. 3. Respiration Disorders—therapy—problems. 4. Respiration Disorders—
therapy—case studies.
WF 18.2 M477r 1997]
RC732.M395 1997
616.2'406—dc21
DNLM/DLC
for Library of Congress   97-3043
                                                                    CIP

RESPIRATORY CARE PEARLS   ISBN 1-56053-204-1

Last digit is the printed number: 9 8 7 6 5 4 3 2 1

THE PEARLS SERIES®

Series Editors

Steven A. Sahn, M.D.
Professor of Medicine
Director, Division of Pulmonary
  and Critical Care Medicine
Medical University of South
  Carolina
Charleston, South Carolina

John E. Heffner, M.D.
Professor of Clinical Medicine
University of Arizona
  Health Sciences Center
Chairman, Academic Internal Medicine
St. Joseph's Hospital and Medical Center
Phoenix, Arizona

The books in The Pearls Series® contain 75–100 case presentations that provide valuable information that is not readily available in standard textbooks. The problem-oriented approach is ideal for self-study and for board review. A brief clinical vignette is presented, including physical examination and laboratory findings, accompanied by a radiograph, EKG, or other pertinent illustration. The reader is encouraged to consider a differential diagnosis and formulate a plan for diagnosis and treatment. The subsequent page discloses the diagnosis, followed by a discussion of the case, clinical pearls, and two or three key references.

CARDIOLOGY PEARLS
Blase A. Carabello, MD, William L. Ballard, MD, and Peter C. Gazes, MD, Medical University of South Carolina, Charleston, South Carolina
1994/233 pages/illustrated/ISBN 0-932883-96-6

CRITICAL CARE PEARLS
Steven A. Sahn, MD, Medical University of South Carolina, Charleston, South Carolina, and **John E. Heffner, MD,** St. Joseph's Hospital and Medical Center, Phoenix, Arizona
1989/300 pages/illustrated/ISBN 0-932883-24-9

INTERNAL MEDICINE PEARLS
Clay B. Marsh, MD, and **Ernest L. Mazzaferri, MD,** The Ohio State University College of Medicine, Columbus, Ohio
1992/300 pages/90 illustrations/ISBN 1-56053-024-3

PULMONARY PEARLS
Steven A. Sahn, MD, Medical University of South Carolina, Charleston, South Carolina, and **John E. Heffner, MD,** St. Joseph's Hospital and Medical Center, Phoenix, Arizona
1988/250 pages/illustrated/ISBN 0-932883-16-8

PULMONARY PEARLS II
Steven A. Sahn, MD, Medical University of South Carolina, Charleston, South Carolina, and **John E. Heffner, MD,** St. Joseph's Hospital and Medical Center, Phoenix, Arizona
1995/300 pages/illustrated/ISBN 1-56053-121-5

RESPIRATORY CARE PEARLS
Frank A. Mazzagatti, MSA, RRT, Leon C. Lebowitz, BA, RRT, Brookdale University Hospital and Medical Center, Brooklyn, New York, and **Neil W. Schluger, MD,** Bellevue Hospital and NYU Medical Center, New York, New York
1997/216 pages/illustrated/ISBN 1-56053-204-1

RHEUMATOLOGY PEARLS
Richard M. Silver, MD, and **Edwin A. Smith, MD,** Medical University of South Carolina, Charleston, South Carolina
1997/192 pages/illustrated/ISBN 1-56053-201-7

TUBERCULOSIS PEARLS
Neil W. Schluger, MD, and **Timothy J. Harkin, MD,** Bellevue Hospital and NYU Medical Center, New York, New York

DEDICATION

To my parents,

   Catherine and Frank Mazzagatti,

      for their love, inspiration, and support.

                              FAM

To my wife,

   Elizabeth R. Lebowitz,

      for her love, understanding, and support;

         and my children,

            Jennifer, Lauren, and Jonathan;

               and in memory of my parents,

                  Ruth and Henry Lebowitz

                              LCL

To the most important people in my life,

   my wife Leona,

      and my children Aaron, Benjamin, and Julia.

                              NWS

CONTENTS

Patient   **Page**

Patient   **Page**

CONTRIBUTORS

Numbers in parentheses refer to cases written or cowritten.

Theresa M. Barrett-Jasensky, MA, RRT
Assistant Professor and Program Director, Respiratory Care Program, Malloy College, Rockville Centre, New York
(12, 40, 43, 66)

Robert R. Fluck, Jr., MS, RRT
Associate Professor and Clinical Coordinator, Department of Cardiorespiratory Sciences, SUNY Health Science Center, Syracuse, New York
(56, 57, 64, 65)

Jay S. Greenspan, MD
Associate Professor of Pediatrics, Director, Division of Neonatology, Thomas Jefferson University, Jefferson Medical College, Philadelphia, Pennsylvania
(29, 30)

George W. Gross, MD
Professor of Radiology and Pediatrics, Thomas Jefferson University, Philadelphia, Pennsylvania; Chairman, Department of Medical Imaging, DuPont Hospital for Children, Wilmington, Delaware
(29, 30)

Robert F. Jasensky, BA, RRT
Clinical Director, Prime Care Medical Supplies, Inc., Flushing, New York
(12, 40, 43, 66)

Brian Kaufman, MD
Assistant Professor of Anesthesiology and Medicine, NYU School of Medicine; Director, Section of Critical Care Medicine, and Associate Medical Director, Surgical Intensive Care Unit, NYU Medical Center, New York, New York
(31, 32)

Stephen J. Lowenstein, MS, RRT
Technical Director, Pulmonary Physiology Laboratory, Lenox Hill Hospital, New York, New York
(39, 41)

Thomas H. Shaffer, PhD
Professor of Physiology and Pediatrics, Director, Respiratory Physiology Section, Temple University School of Medicine, Philadelphia, Pennsylvania
(29, 30)

Robert J. Sparaco, BS, JD, RRT
Associate Professor, Department of Allied Health Sciences, Nassau Community College; Education Coordinator, Respiratory Care Department, NYU Medical Center, New York, New York
(31, 32)

Robert D. Walsh, MD, PhD
Medical Director, AIDS Designated Center, The Brookdale University Hospital and Medical Center, Brooklyn, New York
(68, 73)

Miroslav B. Zotovic, MD
Senior Pulmonary Fellow, Department of Pulmonary Medicine, Lenox Hill Hospital, New York, New York
(39, 41)

FOREWORD

The Pearls Series® developed by Steve Sahn and John Heffner has proved a unique and effective way to teach clinical medicine. In each volume, cases are presented that represent the range of clinical problems relating to the specific topic. With each case, the reader is challenged to create a differential diagnosis and management plan. In the ensuing discussion, important teaching points are brought forward and the reader is left with 3 "pearls" (take-home treasures) that distill the critical points. This problem-oriented format not only brings out important teaching points, but does so in a way that reminds us of the "fun" of clinical medicine. As might be expected, this series has been particularly useful as a problem-oriented board review tool.

Given my enthusiasm for this format, I was delighted to learn that the Pearls Series® was now going to include *Respiratory Care Pearls*, written by Frank Mazzagatti, Leon Lebowitz, and Neil Schluger. Respiratory care is certainly deserving of its own volume given its uniqueness in integrating clinical medicine and technology. Clinicians involved in respiratory care face daily problems requiring expertise in assessment and in formulating a plan of care that often involves complex equipment and life-support systems. Problems thus arise not only in determining the pathophysiologic process but also in setting up, monitoring, and troubleshooting equipment. The Pearls format allows the authors to address these issues by presenting a number of typical clinical problems that the respiratory care clinician faces every day. The assessment and reasoning process that must be applied to these patients is carefully discussed in each. Therapeutic plans and subsequent management issues are developed, and at the end of each discussion the important "take-home pearls" are emphasized.

Respiratory Care Pearls not only brings information but also emphasizes the "fun" of practicing respiratory care. This book is must reading for all serious clinicians involved in respiratory care.

Neil R. MacIntyre, MD
Professor of Medicine
Medical Director, Respiratory Care Services
Duke University Medical Center
Durham, North Carolina

EDITORS' FOREWORD

Clinical problem-solving that results in improved outcome in a seriously ill patient is one of the most gratifying experiences in the practice of medicine. Few areas of medicine present such a steady stream of problem-solving challenges than the management of patients with respiratory insufficiency. Physicians, respiratory therapists, and nurses who care for these patients require a broad range of skills to address the complex medical, surgical, pharmacologic, and emotional needs of their patients. Considering the twin challenges of "managing" sophisticated monitoring equipment and mechanical ventilators, in addition to the patients themselves, respiratory care practitioners are called upon to keep their problem-solving abilities extraordinarily sharp.

Toward this goal, *Respiratory Care Pearls* provides a valuable approach to enhancing clinical skills. In editing this and the other books in the Pearls Series®, we have attempted to develop a consistent format and style that challenge the reader by presenting the salient features of a clinical problem and directing attention to an important question in management. The discussion that follows first reviews the patient's general disorder and then focuses on the unique aspects of the presented patient's condition. Throughout the discussion, aspects of diagnosis and care that are especially important, "cutting edge," or not widely recognized are captured and listed at the end of each discussion as "Clinical Pearls." Finally, so as not to lose sight of our interest in the individual patient, the discussion closes with the clinical outcome of the patient at hand. In the process, student readers beginning their medical careers, residents in training, and experienced respiratory therapists, critical care nurses, and physicians honing their skills will find something of value in each of the patient presentations.

We greatly appreciate the efforts of Frank Mazzagatti, Leon Lebowitz, and Neil Schluger in adding *Respiratory Care Pearls* as the eighth book in the Pearls Series®. As seasoned experts in respiratory care, they have provided us with excellent examples, in these 75 patient presentations with accompanying Pearls, of how astute bedside problem-solving translates into superb clinical care for our patients.

John E. Heffner, MD
Steven A. Sahn, MD
Editors, The Pearls Series®

PREFACE

The field of respiratory care is an ever-changing specialty. Advances in technology and the proliferation of respiratory therapy equipment have made the challenge of caring for these patients increasingly sophisticated and complex. There are very few respiratory texts available to the practicing clinician which synthesize both theory and clinical applications. Our goal in adding *Respiratory Care Pearls* to The Pearls Series® was to provide a primary text to fill that void. The book is intended for respiratory therapists, physicians, fellows, residents, nurses, students, and academicians who find themselves intrigued and challenged by these problems, and who are also responsible for the integration of respiratory care practice into delivery of care to their patients.

We wish to acknowledge the support and help of our colleagues at the Brookdale University Hospital and Medical Center and the New York University Medical Center in the preparation of this volume, and we specifically thank the Departments of Respiratory Therapy, Radiology, Pulmonology, Surgery, Administration, Medical Records, Medical Library, and Medical Photography. We also give special thanks to Boysing A. Samuel, RRT, and Cecelia Fortune.

Frank A. Mazzagatti, RRT
Leon C. Lebowitz, RRT
Neil W. Schluger, MD

PATIENT 1

A 51-year-old man with dyspnea, hypotension, bradycardia, and pulmonary infiltrates

A 51-year-old morbidly obese man was admitted to the emergency department from home with dyspnea, hypotension, and bradycardia. He had suddenly become dyspneic while eating. Past medical history featured severe obesity, chronic obstructive pulmonary disease, cellulitis, and depression. Prehospital emergency care included intravenous access with fluid replacement. Medications included anhydrous theophylline, albuterol, ipratropium, and fluoxetine.

Physical Examination: Temperature 99°; pulse 60; respirations 28; blood pressure 90/palpable. Chest: diffuse rhonchi with bilateral polyphonic wheezes. Cardiac: regular rhythm without murmurs, gallops, or rubs. Abdomen: nontender, without organomegaly. Extremities: no clubbing, cyanosis, or edema. Neurologic: nonfocal.

Laboratory Findings: WBC 11,000/µl, Hct 28%, platelets 360,000/µl. ABG (FiO$_2$ .50), pH 7.07, pCO$_2$ 102 mmHg, pO$_2$ 34 mmHg, HCO$_3^-$ 27 mEq/L, SaO$_2$ 63%. Chest: see radiograph below.

Hospital Course: He was intubated and placed on a Siemens Servo 900C ventilator with the following settings: CMV, V$_t$ 1000 ml, f = 25, FiO$_2$ 1.0 with 16 cm H$_2$O PEEP resulting in a mean airway pressure of 72–82 cm H$_2$O.

Questions: What is the most probable cause of the patient's respiratory failure? What are the criteria for the use of pressure-controlled ventilation?

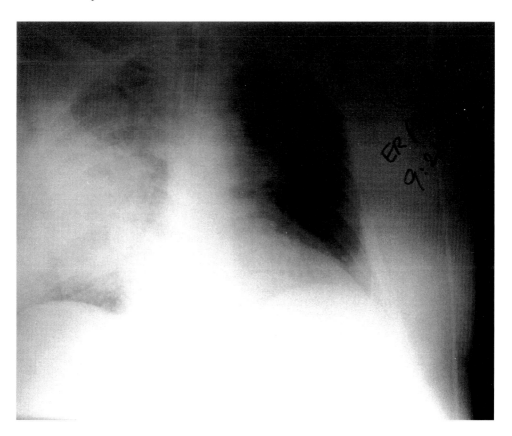

Diagnosis: Aspiration pneumonia–induced ARDS.

Discussion: The adult respiratory distress syndrome (ARDS) comprises a heterogeneous group of disorders which lead to the same pattern of tissue injury in the lung. Refractory hypoxemia, bilateral pulmonary infiltrates, and reduced static effective compliance with preservation of normal pulmonary capillary wedge pressure remain classic diagnostic criteria for ARDS. Though the nature of the original insult can be diverse (trauma, infection, hypotension, immunologic challenge), the tissue response in ARDS is remarkably uniform, demonstrating an influx of inflammatory cells (predominantly, but not exclusively, neutrophils), hyaline membrane formation, hyperplasia of type II pneumocytes, and eventually fibrosis. The physiologic manifestations of ARDS are also uniform despite the underlying insult. Two of these physiologic derangements, severe abnormalities of gas exchange due to ventilation/perfusion mismatching and markedly reduced lung compliance, provide the greatest challenges to artificial respiratory support.

Because of abnormalities of lung compliance, ventilator management of the patient with ARDS is associated with common problems, such as pulmonary barotrauma, that only complicate an already tenuous lung process. It is now clear that excessive lung distention is a major factor in overt barotrauma and that distending volume, not only airway pressure, determines lung injury. Therefore the current approach to ventilatory support incorporates a "lung-protective" strategy for the purpose of supporting gas exchange while avoiding ventilator-induced lung damage.

Because of concerns about barotrauma, several new approaches to mechanical ventilation have been advocated, and there is a rationale for each. **Pressure-controlled ventilation** is a strategy that aims to limit directly the high-inflation pressures and volumes associated with ARDS patients receiving artificial respiratory support. Controlling mean airway pressure and mean alveolar pressure can limit barotrauma related not only to overdistension of the lung as a whole but also to individual alveoli, which may be subject to very different inflation pressures as a result of the inhomogeneity of the ARDS disease process. Indeed, evidence now exists that overinflation of individual alveoli can be associated with worsening lung injury (so-called volutrauma).

In the most common type of pressure-controlled ventilation, the maximal airway pressure is preset, and the delivered tidal volume depends on the difference in pressure between the airway opening and the alveolus at the beginning of ventilation, as well as airway resistance, airway compliance, and the inspiratory time. It is often easiest to employ this mode in a sedated patient, so as to avoid the problem of patient-ventilator dyssynchrony. The major goal is to provide adequate gas exchange, even at the expense of hypercapnia. In fact, one often chooses to allow hypercapnia to develop in this setting as an acceptable consequence of reduced pulmonary pressures. Such a strategy is termed **permissive hypercapnia**, and it is being widely adopted as a ventilatory strategy. (Permissive hypercapnia is a strategy that also may be employed with volume-cycled ventilation, using lower than traditional tidal volumes—for example, 5–8 cc/kg.)

The current patient was ventilated with pressure-controlled ventilation to maintain airway pressures no higher than 35 cm H_2O. Despite this, multisystem organ failure developed and the patient eventually expired after a prolonged hospital course.

Clinical Pearls

1. High airway pressures are associated not only with barotrauma manifested as pneumothorax, but also as worsening lung injury from overdistension of alveoli.

2. Pressure-controlled ventilation is a ventilatory strategy that allows limits to be set on airway pressures, though a guaranteed tidal volume is not delivered.

3. Permissive hypercapnia, often accompanying pressure-controlled ventilation, is an additional strategy that may be used to limit barotrauma.

REFERENCES
1. MacIntyre NR. Minimizing alveolar stretch injury during mechanical ventilation. Respir Care 1996; 41:318–326.
2. Armstrong BW, MacIntyre NR. Pressure-controlled inverse ratio ventilation that avoids air trapping in the adult respiratory distress syndrome. Crit Care Med 1995;23:279–285.
3. Slutsky AS. Mechanical ventilation: ACCP Consensus Statement. Chest 1993;104:1833–1859.

PATIENT 2

A 33-year-old woman with fever, pleuritic chest pain, and progressive dyspnea

A 33-year-old woman with a known history of alcohol and drug abuse was admitted to the intensive care unit with fever, pleuritic chest pain, and cough. She was being treated for an upper respiratory infection when she suddenly developed severe respiratory distress.

Physical Examination: Temperature 100.6°; pulse 110; respirations 24; blood pressure 110/70. Chest: diminished sounds at the bases, without wheezes. Cardiac: regular rate and rhythm, without murmurs or rubs. Abdomen: soft, without organomegaly. Extremities: no cyanosis, clubbing, or edema. Neurologic: alert and oriented, nonfocal.

Laboratory Findings: WBC 24,300/µl, Hct 41%. ABG (40% O_2 face mask): pH 7.37, pCO_2 37 mmHg, pO_2 133 mmHg, HCO_3^- 19 mEq/L, SaO_2 98%. Sputum Gram stain: gram-positive cocci in clusters. Pleural fluid analysis: see table. Chest radiograph (see below): left infiltrate with pleural effusion.

Question: What is the most probable cause of the patient's pleuritic chest pain?

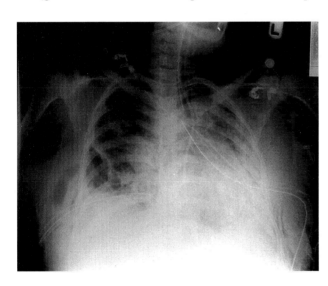

Pleural Fluid Analysis

	Serous, cloudy, yellow
RBC:	850/µl
WBC:	52,000/µl
Polys:	94%
Total Protein:	5.7 g/dl
LDH:	1023 IU/L
Amylase:	20 IU/L
Glucose:	108 mg/dl
pH:	5.0
Cytology:	negative
Culture:	*S. aureus*

Diagnosis: Empyema.

Discussion: Pleural effusion is a common finding in patients with pneumonia, and the treatment of the effusion is determined in large part by the inflammatory characteristics of the pleural fluid. The major differential diagnostic point is to determine whether the fluid represents a true infection of the pleural space (empyema) or is an inflammatory response to the infection in the lung (parapneumonic effusion). Empyema, defined as a **pleural effusion** in which organisms are seen on Gram stain or which has the characteristics of pus (high neutrophil count, low pH), is a condition requiring the same treatment as any closed-space infection—namely, drainage.

A recent review of the etiology of empyema indicated that it often represents a complicated, mixed infection that frequently occurs in patients with underlying illness. In a series of 82 patients, 82% were alcoholic, diabetic, or had an underlying malignancy. Anaerobes were found in the pleural fluid of 28% and multiple organisms were present in 40% of the cases. The level of illness caused by empyema is reflected in the fact that the mean duration of hospital stay in this series was 37 days.

The treatment of **parapneumonic effusion** is somewhat more complicated and controversial. The main concern with non-empyemic inflammatory effusion is that if untreated it will form a thick fibrotic rind or "peel" around the infected lung and leave the patient with a restrictive pulmonary defect. Determining prospectively which parapneumonic effusions will self-absorb and which will require drainage is not always a straightforward process but useful criteria have been suggested. If the pH of the fluid is higher than 7.20, the patient likely has an uncomplicated parapneumonic effusion which will resolve without treatment. Non-empyemic effusion with a pH less than 7.10 is likely to require drainage. Parapneumonic effusion with intermediate pH should be monitored, and repeat thoracentesis should be performed until the clinical course becomes clear.

In treating empyema, drainage traditionally has been achieved through a large-bore thoracostomy tube inserted into the pleural space. However, in the past several years a variety of other approaches have been attempted, and they may be appropriate to use in certain circumstances. It is increasingly recognized that complicated pleural space infections often involve loculated collections of fluid, and these will not be adequately drained by placement without imaging guidance of a chest tube into a fluid pocket. Thus, video-assisted thoracoscopic drainage, with or without debridement and decortication, is an alternative approach to pleural space infection, as is placement of a small-bore catheter under CT scan guidance followed by the instillation of streptokinase or urokinase to break up loculations of fluid and allow drainage. In several reports, these approaches have been associated with excellent results and shortened hospital stays.

Following thoracentesis, the patient in this case underwent placement of a chest tube for drainage of the empyema. Drainage was accomplished without the need for further intervention. The patient responded to antibiotic therapy and was discharged 3 weeks following admission.

Clinical Pearls

1. Patients with fever and pleural effusion should undergo thoracentesis to determine the need for drainage of the pleural space.

2. Organisms seen on Gram stain of pleural fluid or frank pus obtained from the pleural space are indications for chest tube placement. Indeterminate effusions should have follow-up thoracentesis to determine the need for drainage.

3. Alternatives to tube thoracostomy include video-assisted thoracoscopic surgery or placement of a radiographically-guided catheter followed by instillation of a thrombolytic agent to break up loculations.

REFERENCES

1. Landreneau RJ, Keenan RJ, Hazelrigg SR, et al. Thoracoscopy for empyema and hemothorax. Chest 1996;109:18–24.
2. Moulton JS, Benkert RE, Weisiger KH, Chambers JA. Treatment of complicated pleural fluid collections with image-guided drainage and intracavitary urokinase. Chest 1995;108:1252–1259.
3. Sendt W, Forster E, Hau T. Early thoracoscopic debridement and drainage as definite treatment for pleural empyema. Eur J Surg 1995;161:73–76.
4. Heffner J, Brown LK, Barbieri C, DeLeo JM. Pleural fluid chemical analysis in parapneumonic effusions: A meta-analysis. Am J Respir Crit Care Med 1995;151:1700–1708.
5. Strange C, Sahn SA. The clinician's perspective on parapneumonic effusions and empyema. Chest 1993;103:259–261.

PATIENT 3

A 56-year-old woman with dyspnea and general malaise

A 56-year-old woman was brought to the emergency department complaining of difficulty breathing and general weakness for 2 days. Past medical history included chronic obstructive pulmonary disease (COPD) and kyphoscoliosis. Medications included continuous home oxygen, furosemide, ipratropium, albuterol, prednisolone, and theophylline.

Physical Examination: Temperature 99.8°; pulse 100; respirations 28; blood pressure 110/80. Chest: air entry poor, without wheezes. Cor: distant heart sounds, no gallop heard, JVD present. Abdomen: soft, without masses or organomegaly. Extremities: ++ pedal edema. Neurologic: normal.

Laboratory Findings: WBC 8700/μl, Hct 51.7%. Na^+ 135 mEq/L, K^+ 4.8 mEq/L, Cl^- 87 mEq/L. BUN 45 mg/dl, Cr 3.4 mg/dl, Albumin 2.8 g/dl, phosphate 7.2 mg/dl, Mg 1.3 mg/dl, theophylline 6.4 μg/ml. ABG (O_2 2 L/min via nasal cannula): pH 7.21, pCO_2 79 mmHg, pO_2 65 mmHg, HCO_3^- 32 mEq/L, SaO_2 88%. Chest radiograph: large amorphous right pleural calcification in the posterior aspect of the lung with pulmonary vascular congestion and cardiomegaly (see below, left). Spinal radiograph: rotary scoliosis (see below, right).

Questions: What is the most probable cause of the patient's symptoms? How is oxygen best administered to such a patient?

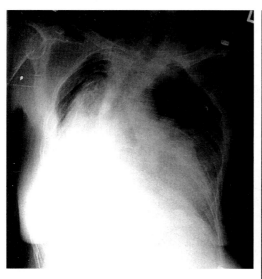 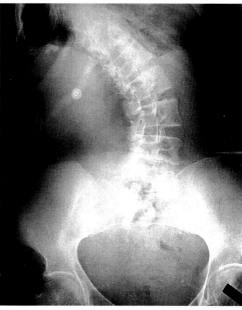

Diagnosis: Acute exacerbation of COPD.

Discussion: Effective management of the patient with COPD must take into account the altered pulmonary physiology that is inherent to the specific disorder, as well as the ventilatory, pharmacological, and nutritional support required to optimize lung function. The anatomic alterations present in the airways of the COPD patient classically include mucosal edema, submucosal gland hypertrophy, bronchospasm, elevation of residual volume, and destruction of the elastic tissues which support the small airways. The functional impairment that is considered the hallmark of this disease group is **expiratory airflow obstruction**, and this obstruction typically is much worse during an acute exacerbation.

In patients with chronic hyperinflation of the lungs, as occurs with severe emphysema, the chest wall becomes distorted, with increased retrosternal air and flattening of the diaphragms (the familiar "barrel chest" configuration). The distortion in chest wall architecture places the respiratory muscles at a significant mechanical disadvantage so that the oxygen cost of breathing (the amount of cardiac output or oxygen consumption devoted to breathing) rises from the 2–5% observed in normals to as high as 15–40%. This places patients with COPD at great risk for respiratory muscle fatigue and respiratory failure.

The restrictive disorder of scoliosis further increases the work of breathing because the spinal deformity and decreased chest wall compliance limit inspiratory volumes, causing reduced spontaneous tidal volumes and an increased breathing rate. Thus, in addition to the usual bronchodilator therapy, simply resting patients with COPD exacerbations often achieves significant beneficial effects by avoiding unnecessary expenditures of energy.

Oxygen therapy in patients with COPD exacerbations must be judiciously applied. It has long been observed that in certain COPD patients oxygen therapy results in steep rises in pCO_2 and an acute respiratory acidosis. These problems were believed to be caused by the extinguishing of the hypoxic ventilatory drive upon which patients with COPD appeared to depend.

However, recent work suggests another, more important, mechanism—namely, a worsening of **ventilation/perfusion (V/Q) mismatching** in response to oxygen. This worsening of V/Q mismatching is probably the most significant factor in the development of hypercapnia after administering oxygen. The Haldane effect, relating to the physical properties of gases in solution also is partly responsible.

Though our understanding of the mechanism behind the development of hypercapnia has changed, the approach to providing oxygen has not. Patients with COPD exacerbation should receive the minimal amount of oxygen necessary to achieve an oxygen saturation of 90%. This is often possible with no more than 0.5 L/min or 1 L/min of oxygen by nasal cannula, but more tightly controlled oxygen therapy can be achieved by delivering 24% or 28% oxygen by a Ventimask. If excess oxygen is delivered and hypercapnia develops, there is often little recourse except intubation and mechanical ventilation, as withdrawal of the excess oxygen will only result in a hypercapnic, acidotic patient who is now more hypoxic than at the time the oxygen was initially added.

The present patient averted endotracheal intubation by receiving nasal BiPAP. Bronchodilators, oxygen, diuretics, and antibiotics were administered, and the patient was discharged home after a 7-day hospital stay.

Clinical Pearls

1. A significant component of respiratory failure during a COPD exacerbation is fatigue of the respiratory muscles, and rest is an underappreciated but important component of therapy.

2. The development of hypercapnia in patients with COPD receiving supplemental oxygen is largely due to a worsening of ventilation/perfusion mismatching; reduction in hypoxic drive plays a much less significant role.

3. Oxygen should be provided to patients with acute hypercapnic respiratory failure in the lowest amount possible to maintain oxygen saturation of 90%.

REFERENCES
1. Polkey MI, Kyroussis D, Hamnegard C-H, Mills GH, et al. Diaphragm strength in chronic obstructive pulmonary disease. Am J Respir Crit Care Med 1996;154:1310–1317.
2. Montes de Oca M, Rassulo J, Celli B. Respiratory muscle and cardiopulmonary function during exercise in very severe COPD. Am J Respir Crit Care Med 1996;154:1284–1289.
3. Hanson CW 3rd, Marshall BE, Frasch HF, Marshall C. Causes of hypercarbia with oxygen therapy in patients with chronic obstructive pulmonary disease. Crit Care Med 1996;24:23–28.
4. Berry RB, Mahutte CK, Kirsch JL, Stansbury DW, et al. Does the hypoxic ventilatory response predict the oxygen-induced falls in ventilation in COPD? Chest 1993;103:820–824.

PATIENT 4

A 52-year-old woman with severe dyspnea, hypotension, and chest pain

A 52-year-old woman with a past medical history of congestive heart failure and hypertension experienced a sudden onset of dyspnea. Paramedics arrived and found the patient hypotensive with frothy sputum. She was transported to the emergency department after initiation of intravenous dopamine (5 μg/kg/min).

Physical Examination: Temperature 98.2°; pulse 110 and irregular; respirations 24 and labored; blood pressure 90/60. Chest: bilateral crackles and rhonchi. Neurologic: cranial nerves intact; alert and oriented, although lethargic.

Laboratory Findings: WBC 11,600/μl, Hct 33.8%, platelets 119,000/μl. Albumin 2.9 g/dl, ALT 122 IU/L, LDH 724 IU/L, CPK 1773 IU/L, BUN 33 mg/dl, Cr 1.8 mg/dl. Sputum: Gram stain revealed few gram-positive cocci. ABG (100% O_2 non-rebreathing mask): pH 7.38 pCO_2 38 mmHg, pO_2 53 mmHg. Chest radiograph (see below): bilateral pulmonary infiltrates. EKG: 2–3 mm ST segment elevation in leads II, III, and aVF.

Hospital Course: The patient was electively intubated and transferred to the cardiac care unit where she was started on dobutamine and a pulmonary artery catheter was inserted demonstrating the following hemodynamics: PAS/PAD 46/28 mmHg with mean PAP 34 mmHg, PAOP 26 mmHg, CO 5.9 L/min, and CI 3.1 L/min/m^2.

Questions: What is the etiology of the patient's respiratory failure? How can the hemodynamics found during right heart catheterization be explained?

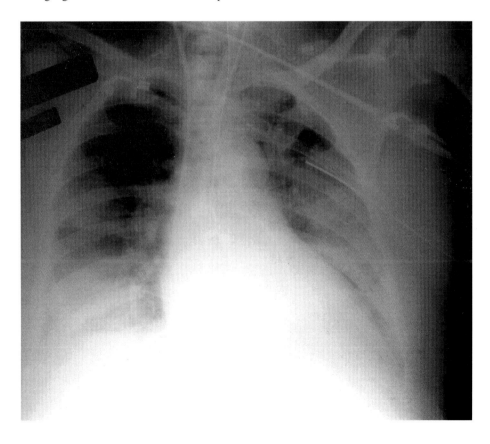

Diagnosis: Cardiogenic pulmonary edema caused by an acute myocardial infarction.

Discussion: This patient presented with the classic signs and symptoms of "flash" pulmonary edema followed by cardiogenic shock: the abrupt onset of severe dyspnea followed by production of pink frothy sputum and hypotension. This condition typically is caused by acute myocardial insufficiency. The patient's physical examination was notable for rales and rhonchi, and chest radiograph demonstrated diffuse infiltrates characteristic of pulmonary edema. Although left ventricular dysfunction is the most common cause of cardiogenic pulmonary edema, other entities can result in a similar clinical presentation. These states include severe volume overload (seen in patients with renal insufficiency, for example), mechanical obstruction of the left atrium (due to left atrial myxoma), pulmonary venous hypertension, or valvular heart disease. More than one factor may contribute, as in the case of pregnancy (a physiologic state associated with increased circulating blood volume) occurring in a woman with mitral stenosis leading to pulmonary edema.

Although a cardiac cause of this patient's pulmonary edema was suggested strongly by her history of congestive heart failure and hypertension, it was important to confirm the diagnosis with an electrocardiogram and right heart catheterization. EKG was diagnostic of an acute inferior wall myocardial infarction; right heart catheterization confirmed an elevated pulmonary capillary wedge pressure, or more accurately, pulmonary artery occlusion pressure. The relatively normal cardiac output and cardiac index measured in this patient were undoubtedly related to the inotropic and pressor support she was receiving, as hypotension and pulmonary edema associated with cardiac failure are usually seen in conjunction with a cardiac index of less than 2.2 L/min/m^2.

In patients such as this with respiratory failure of cardiac etiology, primary therapy is aimed at treating the patient's heart disease while providing adequate respiratory support until eventual recovery. Mortality in cardiogenic pulmonary edema with shock remains extremely high, approaching 60–80% in most series. Treating myocardial ischemia through revascularization with thrombolytic therapy, angioplasty, or coronary artery bypass surgery may be lifesaving. Reducing myocardial work, by decreasing both preload and afterload, can be achieved with vasoactive agents and diuresis, though hypotension often limits this approach. The addition of inotropes such as dobutamine may transiently increase cardiac output, but this strategy has a cost as well because it increases myocardial oxygen consumption. Intra-aortic balloon counterpulsation, the most effective means of reducing afterload, may be a bridge to revascularization, as may newer left ventricular assist devices.

The mechanism of hypoxia in patients with cardiogenic pulmonary edema involves a combination of shunt, ventilation-perfusion mismatching due to regional atelectasis, and perhaps decreased diffusing capacity because of interstitial edema. Positive-pressure ventilation with addition of positive end-expiratory pressure (PEEP) increases oxygenation primarily by recruiting additional alveoli for gas exchange. Positive-pressure ventilation also helps to overcome the increased work of breathing caused by the decreased lung compliance typical of pulmonary edema states. Though PEEP may decrease venous return at high levels and drop preload, it does not reduce total lung water.

The patient in this case was treated with furosemide and nitroglycerin for preload reduction, dobutamine for inotropy, and mechanical ventilation for respiratory support. Her hypoxemia and pulmonary edema improved after 3 days and she was weaned from the ventilator.

Clinical Pearls

1. Right heart catheterization can aid in distinguishing cardiogenic from noncardiogenic pulmonary edema. Distinguishing these entities on the basis of chest radiographs is difficult.

2. Positive-pressure ventilation decreases left ventricular preload by raising mean intrathoracic pressure and may improve gas exchange by improving cardiac function and reducing pulmonary edema.

3. Although inotropes, pressors, and intraortic counterpulsation devices may all improve left ventricular function and improve outcome in cardiogenic shock, revascularization and myocardial salvage remain the best strategies for improving the patient's ultimate prognosis.

REFERENCES

1. Grella RD, Becker RC. Cardiogenic shock complicating coronary artery disease: Diagnosis, treatment, and management. Curr Probl Cardiol 1994;19(12):699–742.
2. Shephard JN, Brecker SJ, Evans TW. Bedside assessment of myocardial performance in the critically ill. Intens Care Med 1994;20(7):513–521.
3. Wickerts CJ, Berg B, Blomqvist H. Influence of positive end-expiratory pressure on extravascular lung water during the formation of experimental hydrostatic pulmonary oedema. Acta Anaesthesiol Scand 1992;36(4):309–317.

PATIENT 5

A 51-year-old man with respiratory distress, fever, and bilateral interstitial infiltrates

A 51-year-old man with a past medical history of AIDS, hypertension, hepatic encephalopathy, and coagulopathy was brought to the emergency department with respiratory distress, fever, and bilateral interstitial infiltrates. He was intubated for progressively worsening hypoxemia with fatigue.

Physical Examination: Temperature 101.3°; pulse 90; respirations 32 and labored; blood pressure 130/90; weight 67.3 kg. Chest: bilateral rhonchi. Abdomen: distended. Neurologic: responsive to painful stimuli.

Laboratory Findings: WBC 12,500/µl. Na^+ 142 mEq/L, K^+ 3.6 mEq/L, Cl^- 112 mEq/L, HCO_3^- 17 MEq/L, TCO_2 13 mEq/L. BUN 132 mg/dl, Cr 3.9 mg/dl. Alk phos 211 IU/L, amylase 721 IU/L, AST 79 IU/L, GGT 515 IU/L, LDH 386 IU/L, albumin 1.8 g/dl, total bilirubin 1.3 mg/dl. PT 11.9 sec, PTT 27.7 sec, $CD4^+$ 50 cells/mm^3. ABG (FiO_2 0.50, by facemask): pH 7.36, pCO_2 30 mmHg, pO_2 48 mmHg, SaO_2 83%. Chest radiograph (see below): bilateral interstitial infiltrates.

Hospital Course: The patient was placed on a Siemens Servo 900C ventilator with the following settings: volume control, V_t 700 ml, f = 20, FiO_2 .75, with 7 cm H_2O of PEEP. Repeat ABG: pH 7.50, pCO_2 28 mmHg, pO_2 73 mmHg, HCO_3^- 22 mEq/L, SaO_2 96%.

Question: What is the most likely diagnosis in this patient?

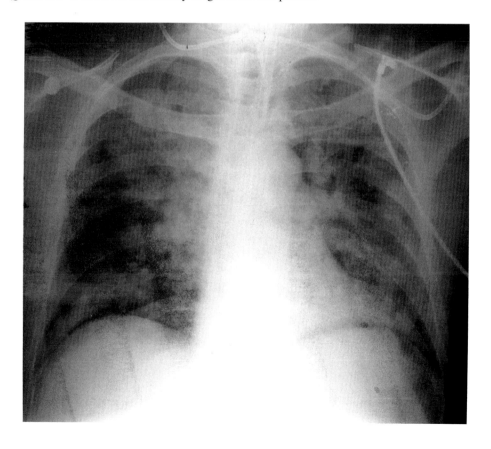

Diagnosis: Acute respiratory failure due to *Pneumocystis carinii* pneumonia (PCP).

Discussion: Pulmonary complications of the acquired immunodeficiency syndrome (AIDS) are the most substantial causes of morbidity and mortality resulting from infection with the human immunodeficiency virus (HIV). The recently completed Pulmonary Complications of AIDS Study, a multicenter investigation conducted over several years, has clearly established the type and pattern of lung disease seen in these patients. It is now recognized that the most common **pulmonary complications of AIDS** are episodes of bronchitis and bacterial pneumonia. These generally occur somewhat earlier in the course of HIV infection, when the T-helper (CD4+) cell count is still relatively high, usually greater than 500/µl. In this clinical stage of the disease, repeated episodes of bronchitis and pneumonia, often caused by somewhat less common, community-acquired pathogens such as *Pseudomonas aeruginosa*, are typical.

When the CD4+ cell count falls below 200/µl, disease due to opportunistic pathogens is frequent and begins to dominate the clinical syndrome. Common opportunistic pathogens causing pulmonary disease at this stage of HIV infection include *Pneumocystis carinii*, *Mycobacterium tuberculosis*, *Histoplasma capsulatum*, *Cryptococcus neoformans*, and, on occasion, cytomegalovirus. Pulmonary disease caused by more unusual organisms, such as *Rhodococcus equi* and *Toxoplasma gondii*, has also been reported. However, by far the most serious opportunist in this setting is *Pneumocystis carinii*.

Once thought to be a protozoan, but now classified by most as a fungus, *Pneumocystis carinii* for years has been known to cause an interstitial pneumonitis in severely debilitated hosts, such as severely malnourished children or patients receiving chemotherapy for lymphomas and leukemias. However, the number of cases of PCP rose dramatically with the onset of the AIDS epidemic. Indeed, AIDS was first recognized when the Centers for Disease Control noted an abnormally large number of requests for anti-PCP drugs. There has been some debate about whether cases of PCP represent reactivation of latent organisms residing in a previously healthy host or whether disease occurs as a result of recent transmission and infection. Although this is still an unresolved question, it is not the practice of most physicians to place patients with PCP in respiratory isolation.

As a complication of AIDS, PCP clinically presents insidiously, with slowly increasing dyspnea and a nonproductive cough. Patients typically have less than 200 CD4+ cells/µl. The chest radiograph typically shows diffuse interstitial infiltrates which can progress to diffuse air-space consolidation and ARDS if untreated. Cystic lesions and pneumothorax have been increasingly recognized. Pleural effusions and lymphadenopathy are rare.

Diagnosis of PCP can be established in a number of ways. Least invasive is staining of an induced sputum sample with methenamine silver, toluidine blue, or equivalent. If sputum is properly collected and stained, the diagnostic yield can be as high as 80%. Failing this, bronchoalveolar lavage is diagnostic in at least 90% of cases; transbronchial biopsy further increases the yield, demonstrating characteristic granular eosinophilic material (identical to that seen in alveolar proteinosis) filling alveolar spaces, as well as characteristic cysts of the organism.

First-line treatment of PCP is with trimethoprim-sulfamethoxazole (TMP-SMX). Pentamidine and trimetrexate are used in sulfa intolerant patients. In patients who present with severe disease (A-a gradient > 30 mmHg or pO_2 < 70 mmHg, on room air) steroids should be used, as this has clearly been shown to reduce mortality. Patients who have been appropriately treated but who progress to respiratory failure have an extremely poor prognosis, and institution of mechanical ventilation is often futile in this setting. For this reason it is important to remember that **prophylactic therapy with TMP-SMX**, instituted at CD4+ cell counts below 250/µl, dramatically reduces the incidence of PCP, and should be used in all patients.

The patient presented in this case worsened and finally succumbed to his pneumonia.

Clinical Pearls

1. Pulmonary complications of AIDS are related to the underlying level of immunosuppression, with *Pneumocystis carinii* pneumonia (PCP) most common at CD4$^+$ levels less than 200/μl.

2. Adjunctive therapy with corticosteroids should be initiated in patients with PCP who present with an A-a gradient > 30 mmHg or a pO$_2$ < 70 mmHg, on room air.

3. Outcome in patients with PCP and respiratory failure is poor, underscoring the need for prophylactic therapy and prompt diagnosis and treatment of suspected cases.

REFERENCES

1. Fernandez P, Torres A, Miro JM, et al. Prognostic factors influencing the outcome in *Pneumocystis carinii* pneumonia in patients with AIDS. Thorax 1995;50:668–671.
2. Bozette SA, Finkelstein DM, Spector SA, et al. A randomized trial of three antipneumocystis agents in patients with advanced human immunodeficiency virus infection. N Engl J Med 1995;332:693–699.
3. Hirschtick RE, Glassroth J, Jordan MC, et al. Bacterial pneumonia in persons infected with the human immunodeficiency virus. N Engl J Med 1995;333:845–851.
4. Shelhamer JH, Toews GB, Masur H, et al. Respiratory disease in the immunosuppressed patient. Ann Intern Med 1992;117:415–431.
5. Sepkowitz KA, Telzak EE, Gold JW, et al. Pneumothorax in AIDS. Ann Intern Med 1991;114:455–459.

PATIENT 6

A 2-year-old girl with a history of fever, cold, and dyspnea for 3 days

A 2-year-old girl with a history of asthma was evaluated for a 3-day history of fever, coryza, and dyspnea. She had been discharged 1 week earlier from another hospital where she had been treated for an upper respiratory infection. The mother had failed to fill the antibiotic prescription provided at discharge. The patient was brought to the emergency department when her breathing became markedly worse.

Physical Examination: Temperature 102.2°; pulse 126; respirations 30; blood pressure 112/77; weight 10 kg. Chest: bilateral breath sounds with wheezes and basilar crackles. Cardiac: normal S_1 and S_2, no murmur. Neurologic: alert, active, no sensory deficit.

Laboratory Findings: WBC 23,000/μl, Hct 38.6%. Na^+ 122 mEq/L, K^+ 3.3 mEq/L, Cl^- 92 mEq/L, HCO_3^- 35 mEq/L, TCO_2 33 mEq/L. Glucose 97 mg/dl, BUN 4 mg/dl, theophylline 5.1 μg/ml. ABG (FiO_2 0.50): pH 7.07, pCO_2 120 mmHg, pO_2 228 mmHg, SaO_2 99%. Chest radiograph (see below): right middle and lower lobe infiltrates.

Hospital Course: The patient was intubated and started on cefuroxime, aminophylline, albuterol, methylprednisolone, and acetaminophen. She was placed on a Siemens Servo 900C ventilator with the following settings: volume control, V_t 150 ml, f = 30, FiO_2 = .50. Peak airway pressures were in excess of 70 cm H_2O and tidal volume losses of 50 ml were observed.

Questions: What is the diagnosis? What are the likely triggers to this patient's illness?

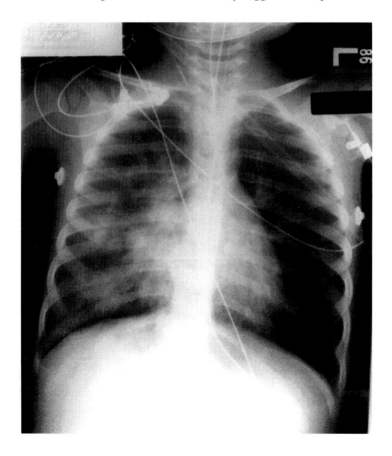

Diagnosis: Status asthmaticus complicated by pneumonia.

Discussion: Asthma is a common but potentially severe respiratory illness that affects many different age groups, including young children. Airway hyperresponsiveness, defined as reversible narrowing of the airways in response to any one of a number of triggers, including but not limited to methacholine, histamine, cold air, exercise, hyperventilation, and allergens, is a frequent finding in the pediatric age group. A study in Australia found that by the age of eight, 8% of children had features of airway hyperresponsiveness and symptoms of asthma. Not all of these children will go on to develop lifelong asthma, and a number of children will have only one or two episodes of wheezing in their lifetime. For this reason, many pediatricians prefer to avoid the label "asthma" and instead apply the diagnosis "hyperreactive airway disease" until symptoms are recurrent over several episodes.

Typically, those children with more severe episodes of wheezing and productive cough are at greater risk for developing lifelong asthma. A recent study provided 25-year follow-up data on children diagnosed as having asthma, wheezing in the presence of an acute respiratory illness, or no respiratory symptoms at all. Though persistent episodes of wheezing occurred in both of the first two groups, individuals who had wheezing only with respiratory infections in childhood were far less likely to go on to develop persistent asthma later in life.

The relationship between allergy and asthma remains a source of controversy, but there is no doubt that allergy must play a significant role in childhood wheezing episodes. In fact, evidence shows that early exposure to mite and/or cockroach antigens in high quantities plays a role in subsequent development of airway hyperresponsiveness. These allergens are ubiquitous, especially in urban areas where the incidence of asthma seems to be rising most quickly. A recent study of children living in metropolitan Washington, D.C. found that 60% were sensitive to cockroach allergen and 72% had allergy to dust mites. Other factors associated with childhood asthma include early exposure to tobacco smoke, including *in utero* exposure.

The role of infection in asthma exacerbation remains unclear. It is well known that adenovirus infections can cause severe respiratory bronchiolitis in children, but the association between these infections and persistent airway obstruction is not firmly established. Recently, adenovirus capsid antigen was found to be present in 91% of the bronchoalveolar lavage fluid in a group of children with obstruction refractory to bronchodilators and corticosteroids. Follow-up studies of a limited number of subjects showed antigen persistence and the presence of virus in BAL fluid. Control children without persistent asthma showed no evidence of virus. On the other hand, there is no evidence to suggest that childhood wheezing is associated with bacterial infections, despite the fact that in this case bacterial pneumonia appeared to be the trigger to the patient's asthma exacerbation and respiratory failure.

Although management of asthma in children is slightly different from management in adults (with the former relying more on drugs such as cromolyn sodium and less on high doses of inhaled corticosteroids), treatment of status asthmaticus is similar for both. This patient received bronchodilator therapy and corticosteroids for their antiinflammatory effect, as well as antibiotics for presumed pneumonia. Ventilator management of a patient with status asthmaticus, discussed in detail elsewhere in this volume, is difficult because of the dangers of dynamic hyperinflation or auto positive end-expiratory pressure, and great care must also be taken to avoid barotrauma.

The patient in this case responded to therapy with the above medications and was successfully extubated and discharged from the hospital.

Clinical Pearls

1. Airway hyperreactivity is common in young children and is not always associated with the development of asthma in later life.

2. Environmental factors such as dust mites, cockroaches, and tobacco smoke are important triggers of wheezing in children.

3. Infections with respiratory viruses such as adenovirus are associated with clinical asthma, though a cause and effect relationship has not been established. Most exacerbations are not due to bacterial infections.

REFERENCES

1. Malveaux FJ, Fletcher-Vincent SA. Environmental risk factors of childhood asthma in urban centers. Environ Health Perspect 1995;103(S)6:59–62.
2. Godden DJ, Ross S, Abdalla M, et al. Outcome of wheeze in childhood: Symptoms and pulmonary function 25 years later. Am J Respir Crit Care Med 1994;149:106–112.
3. Macek V, Sorli J, Kopriva S, Marin J. Persistent adenoviral infection and chronic airway obstruction in children. Am J Respir Crit Care Med 1994;150:7–10.
4. Cox RC, Barker GA, Bohn DJ. Efficacy, results and complications of mechanical ventilation in children with status asthmaticus. Ped Pulmonol 1991;11:120–126.
5. Montgomery GL, Tepper RS. Changes in airway reactivity with age in normal infants and young children. Am Rev Respir Dis 1990;142:1372–1376.

PATIENT 7

A 54-year-old man with a head injury due to a fall from a ladder

A 54-year-old man reportedly fell approximately 15 feet from a ladder and was brought to the emergency department by paramedics. He landed head first, face down with the point of impact being his forehead. Prehospital care included spinal immobilization, establishment of large bore intravenous access, and manual ventilation with a bag-valve mask. Past medical history was unavailable at the time of admission.

Physical Examination: Temperature 100.8°; pulse 120 initially, with gradual decrease in rate; respirations assisted; blood pressure 70/palpation. HEENT: active hemorrhage from the nose and mouth with palpable midface fractures; left eye swollen and proptotic. Chest: bilateral, symetrically decreased breath sounds. Neurologic: unresponsive with a Glasgow Coma Scale score of 3. Skin: multiple lacerations on the face and forehead; right pupil measured 4 mm and sluggish.

Laboratory Findings: Arterial blood gas (FiO_2 1.0): pH 7.21, pCO_2 37 mmHg, pO_2 102 mmHg, HCO_3^- 15 mEq/L, SaO_2 96%. Head CT (see below): diffuse axonal head injury.

Question: What are the principles of respiratory management in a patient with severe head trauma and multiple bodily injuries?

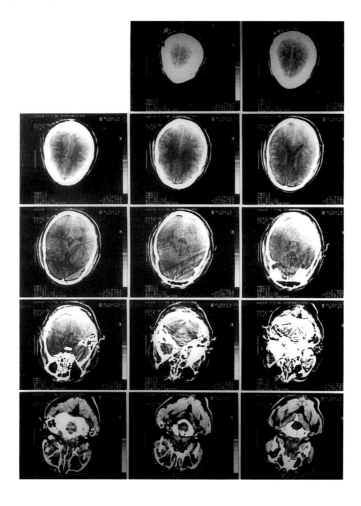

Answer/Discussion: The multiply-injured patient with head trauma presents several challenges to the respiratory physician and therapist. These challenges include attempts to prevent complications arising from an altered sensorium, such as aspiration of gastric contents, as well as efforts to provide direct therapeutic benefit to the injured brain by strategies such as active hyperventilation.

The need to protect a brain-injured patient with a diminished level of consciousness from aspiration and passive upper airway obstruction is an obvious indication for **endotracheal intubation**. However, the possibility of cervical injury and the chance of harming the patient through manipulation of the spine must be considered. If significant cervical injury seems to be present, but the patient's diminished level of consciousness makes intubation the preferred strategy for management, emergency cricothyroidotomy is the best route for protecting the airway. This technique is not without complications, however (including the possibility of damaging vertically oriented arteries and veins in the area of the incision), and may be associated with long-term problems such as scarring and damage to the vocal cords. For these reasons, when an emergency cricothyroidotomy is performed in the field, it is good practice to convert the incision to a standard tracheostomy when the patient stabilizes.

Once the patient has been safely intubated, consideration turns to the best strategy for ventilation in the setting of brain injury. A major focus has always been **hyperventilation** aimed at reducing intracranial pressure to protect the brain from further injury. The mechanism by which hyperventilation may protect the brain is somewhat more complex than is generally appreciated. It is known that reducing arterial CO_2 tension leads to cerebral vasoconstriction, decreased cerebral blood volume, and finally decreased intracranial pressure. Recent evidence also suggests that glucose uptake by the brain may improve with hyperventilation. However, a severely brain-injured patient may have impairment of these reflexes directly due to brain injury or because of accompanying hypotension and hypoxemia. (For this reason, provision of adequate oxygen delivery is a principle of therapy in these circumstances that should not be overlooked.) Most neurosurgical authorities recommend a target CO_2 tension of 25–30 mmHg, and a recent survey of neurosurgical trauma units indicates that over 80% of physicians surveyed use hyperventilation as an *initial* therapeutic approach in patients with closed head injury.

Prolonged hyperventilation is controversial because of concerns about worsening regional brain perfusion despite the beneficial effects of lower overall intracranial pressure. Lowering CO_2 tension below 25–30 mmHg for prolonged periods may be associated with such severe vasoconstriction that cerebral oxygen delivery falls to dangerously low levels, worsening rather than ameliorating brain injury. For this reason, some have advocated the use of cerebral blood flow monitors and/or jugular bulb venous oxygen saturation monitors as guides to proper therapy.

Hyperventilation should be regarded as an initial therapeutic modality which most likely is beneficial only for the first several hours after injury. Continuing hyperventilation beyond a day or two is unlikely to have further ameliorative effects and may be harmful. If the patient shows signs of increasing intracranial pressure (hypotension, bradycardia, loss of reflexes associated with midbrain function) despite hyperventilation into the target zone for CO_2 tension, more definitive therapy should be employed.

For the patient in this case, oral endotracheal intubation was attempted, without success. The airway was established through emergency cricothyroidotomy and the patient was placed on a ventilator with the following settings: V_t 800 ml, f = 24 CMV, FiO_2 1.0. Bilateral chest tubes were inserted, and peritoneal lavage was performed. A central intravenous catheter was inserted for rapid volume replacement. Thirty minutes after admission the patient became bradycardic, then asystolic, and expired.

Clinical Pearls

1. Patients with severe head and neck injuries may require endotracheal intubation for provision of adequate oxygenation and protection of the upper airway from aspiration. Emergency cricothyroidotomy often is the preferred approach because of the potential for worsening a cervical spine injury with trans-laryngeal intubation.

2. Hyperventilation initially may have beneficial effects on intracerebral pressure and glucose uptake by the brain, but prolonged or excessive hyperventilation may be associated with worsening regional brain ischemia and worse outcome.

3. Provision of adequate oxygen delivery to the brain is an often overlooked but essential component in the management of the trauma patient.

REFERENCES

1. Cruz J. An additional therapeutic effect of adequate hyperventilation in acute severe brain trauma: Normalization of cerebral glucose uptake. J Neurosurg 1995;82:379–385.
2. Marion DW, Firlik A, McLaughlin MR. Hyperventilation therapy for severe traumatic brain injury. New Horiz 1995;3:439–447.
3. Rosner MJ, Rosner SD, Johnson AH. Cerebral perfusion pressure: Management protocol and clinical results. J Neurosurg 1995;83:949–962.
4. Ghajar J, Hariri RJ, Narayan RK, Iacono LA, et al. Survey of critical care management or comatose, head-injured patients in the United States. Crit Care Med 1995;23:560–567.
5. Pepe PE, Zacharia BS, Chandra NC. Invasive airway techniques in resuscitation. Ann Emerg Med 1993;22(part 2):393–403.

PATIENT 8

An 81-year-old man with increasing lethargy, dyspnea, and pulmonary infiltrates

An 81-year-old man was brought to the emergency department complaining of increasing lethargy and shortness of breath. The patient had daily production of a large amount of yellow sputum for the previous 5 years. His sputum production had increased markedly recently. Medications included sustained release theophylline, prednisone, furosemide, and methyldopa. The patient was intubated because of marked respiratory distress.

Physical Examination: Temperature 100.7°; pulse 90; respirations 20; blood pressure 100/60; weight 45.9 kg; height 68 inches. Chest: bilateral movement with equal air entry, no adventitious breath sounds, resonant over all lung fields. Cardiac: normal. Neurologic: lethargic but oriented, nonfocal. Skin: poor turgor, mild pedal edema. Extremities: no cyanosis or clubbing.

Laboratory Findings: WBC 33,000/μl, Hct 29.5%. Na^+ 131 mEq/L, K^+ 3.5 mEq/L, Cl^- 89 mEq/L, HCO_3^- 27 mEq/L. BUN 26 mg/dl, Cr 1.2 mg/dl, theophylline 20.6 μg/ml. ABG (FiO_2 0.50): pH 7.07, pCO_2 94 mmHg, pO_2 59 mmHg, SaO_2 77%. Chest radiograph (see below): right upper lobe infiltrate.

Question: What is the underlying etiology of the patient's ventilatory failure?

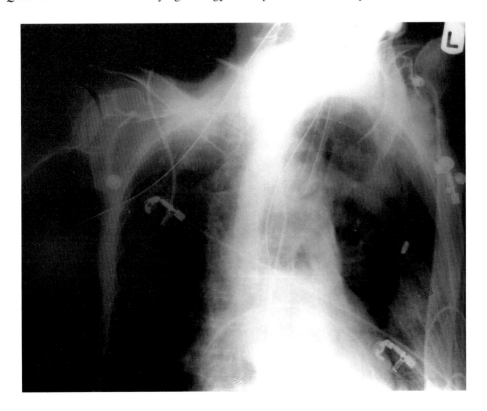

Diagnosis: Bronchiectasis complicated by acute pneumonia and respiratory failure.

Discussion: Bronchiectasis is an abnormal and generally permanent dilatation of the bronchi caused by destruction of elastic and muscular layers of the airway wall. In patients with bronchiectasis, this destruction affects the medium-sized airways, namely those with a diameter of 2 mm or more. The damage can be demonstrated clearly with CT scanning, which has largely replaced bronchography for diagnosing this disease. Though on a gross anatomic basis bronchiectasis can be classified into types such as cylindrical, varicose, and saccular (or cystic), the clinical features of these types are not sufficiently different to make such classifications important in day-to-day management or assessment of patients.

The destruction of the elastic and muscular elements of the medium-sized bronchi is generally assumed to be the result of an **inflammatory process** in most cases, as neutrophils release elastases and other proteolytic enzymes, and other inflammatory cells release a number of cytokines that can add to tissue injury and destruction. Historically, most cases of bronchiectasis are the result of severe pulmonary infections, such as tuberculosis or bacterial or viral pneumonias—a fact that reflects the importance of inflammation in producing this disease.

In industrialized countries, the incidence of bronchiectasis has decreased as pulmonary infections have become more easily treated or prevented, and a number of other, though less common, causes of bronchiectasis are now recognized, including longstanding bronchial obstruction (including the right middle lobe syndrome), cystic fibrosis, the immotile cilia syndrome, primary ciliary dyskinesia, allergic bronchopulmonary aspergillosis, a variety of immunodeficiency states such as IgA and IgG subclass deficiency, alpha-1-antitrypsin deficiency, bronchopulmonary sequestration, and other rare disorders such as the yellow-nail syndrome, tracheobronchomegaly (Mounier-Kuhn syndrome), and unilateral hyperlucent lung syndrome (Swyer-James syndrome). As some of these diseases have specific treatments available (such as steroids for allergic bronchopulmonary aspergillosis), it is important to work through the differential diagnosis when initially evaluating a patient with bronchiectasis.

Regardless of the underlying cause, the common clinical feature and hallmark of bronchiectasis is an inability to clear **respiratory tract secretions**, resulting in chronic production of purulent sputum and predisposition to repeated episodes of pneumonia, which can be complicated by the development of empyema and lung abscess. Because of this, management of patients with bronchiectasis is aimed at reducing secretions and aggressively treating exacerbations of the illness that are caused by infection. Antibiotic therapy is a mainstay of treatment and should be guided by the flora known to colonize the patient's respiratory tract. These organisms may include tenacious, gram-negative bacteria such as *Pseudomonas aeruginosa*. Rotating antibiotics, given for the first few days of each month, is a strategy employed by many, though it is not clear that this approach has a clear advantage over treating only definite exacerbations.

A variety of chest physical therapy techniques, such as postural drainage, cupping and clapping, the use of humidified air, and the use of mucolytic agents such as n-acetylcysteine, have also been advocated for patients with bronchiectasis. However, there is little evidence that nebulized n-acetylcysteine has any true benefit in these patients, and it may actually cause bronchoconstriction in patients so predisposed. Vaccination against pneumococcal pneumonia and influenza should also be given. For patients with very localized bronchiectasis and significant and recurrent symptoms and exacerbations, surgical resection may be curative.

The present patient had developed a severe pneumonia with respiratory failure and required mechanical ventilatory support. Despite the use of vigorous pulmonary toilet, including postural drainage and chest physical therapy as tolerated, aminophylline, beta-adrenergic agents, and antibiotics, the patient's condition deteriorated and he died on the seventh hospital day.

Clinical Pearls

1. Patients with chronic production of purulent sputum should have a diagnostic evaluation for bronchiectasis, a condition that can be difficult to distinguish clinically from chronic bronchitis. The causes of bronchiectasis are diverse, and the spectrum of disease has changed in the antibiotic era.

2. Complications of bronchiectasis include severe pneumonia, empyema, lung abscess, and hemoptysis. Early and aggressive treatment of infectious exacerbations may ameliorate these complications.

3. Antibiotic therapy of exacerbations should be guided by knowledge of the patient's colonizing respiratory tract flora as well as infections prevalent in the community.

REFERENCES

1. Nicotra MB, Rivera M, Dale AM, et al. Clinical, pathophysiologic, and microbiologic characterization of bronchiectasis in an aging cohort. Chest 1995;108:955–961.
2. Ip M, Shum D, Lauder I, Lam WK, et al. Effect of antibiotics on sputum inflammatory contents in acute exacerbations of bronchiectasis. Respir Med 1993;87:449–454.
3. Ip M, Lauder IJ, Wonh WY, et al. Multivariate analysis of factors affecting pulmonary function in bronchiectasis. Respir Med 1993;60:45–50.
4. Conway SH, Fleming JS, Perring S, et al. Humidification as an adjunct to chest physiotherapy in aiding tracheo-bronchial clearance in patients with bronchiectasis. Respir Med 1992;86:109–114.

PATIENT 9

**A 59-year-old man with hypotension and unresponsiveness
after ingestion of pine oil**

A 59-year-old resident of a chronic care facility was brought to the emergency department after having been intubated in the field by EMS when found unresponsive with an empty bottle of liquid cleaner (Pine Sol) beside him. His past medical history included coronary artery disease, hypertension, gout, and a psychiatric disturbance. It was suspected that he ingested the whole bottle (32 ounces) of household cleaner in an attempt to commit suicide. Other medications he was taking included cholestyramine, nifedipine, allopurinol, clonazepam, fluphenazine, and benztropine.

Physical Examination: Temperature 97.2°; pulse 60; respirations assisted; blood pressure 86/palpation. Chest: clear. Neurologic: unresponsive except to painful stimuli; pupils 3 mm, responsive bilaterally. A pungent material was suctioned from the oropharynx.

Laboratory Findings: BUN 59 mg/dl, Cr 4.6 mg/dl, total bilirubin 3.1 mg/dl. Ca 8.7 mg/dl, phosphate 6.5 mg/dl, amylase 192 IU/L. ABG (FiO$_2$ 1.0): pH 7.34, pCO$_2$ 32 mmHg, pO$_2$ 389 mmHg, HCO$_3^-$ 17 mEq/L, SaO$_2$ 99%. Anion gap: normal. Chest radiograph: see below.

Questions: What is the most likely diagnosis for this patient? What general approaches should be used in the management of this patient?

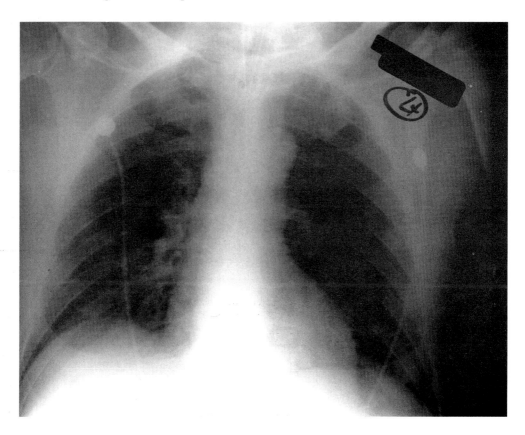

Diagnosis: Pine oil aspiration and toxic ingestion.

Discussion: The management of the poisoned patient is a medical challenge often made more difficult by a lack of information regarding the exact nature of the ingestion. Even for cases such as this one, in which an apparent offending agent is found, it can be a serious error to assume that no additional substances were consumed. Consider the patient's prescription drugs and also easily obtainable, over-the-counter preparations. Once a specific agent has been identified, most toxic ingestions do not require specific therapeutic interventions. Most attention should be paid to providing adequate supportive therapy while eliminating the toxin from the patient's stomach, if possible.

Basic principles of management of poisoned patients begin with the ABCs: **airway, breathing**, and **circulation**. Endotracheal intubation and mechanical ventilation for patients with depressed respiration or risk of aspiration, establishment of intravenous access, and infusion of normal saline for hypotension (a much more common consequence of ingestion than hypertension) are initial steps applicable to *all* patients—regardless of the toxin ingested. Assessment of serum glucose and electrolytes, arterial blood gas analysis, and cardiac monitoring are also routine.

Prevention of further absorption of an ingested substance can be addressed by two mechanisms: direct evacuation of the stomach through gastric lavage or induction of emesis, or absorption by activated charcoal of any remaining toxins. Both of these approaches have implications for respiratory care and prevention of aspiration. At present, induction of emesis with ipecac is less frequent than in the past, and this procedure is rarely used in adult patients at all. It should never be used when there is a concern about ingestion of a caustic substance such as lye, and it should also be avoided in patients with abnormal levels of consciousness or who are at risk for seizures because of possible aspiration.

A similar risk of aspiration may occur with the placement of an orogastric tube for gastric lavage, and if there is any question of altered consciousness, patients should be intubated for airway protection prior to initiation of gastric lavage with a large bore orogastric tube. Indeed, chemical aspiration following toxin ingestion is one of the most dangerous complications that can ensue, and it can lead to the development of adult respiratory distress syndrome. Overall, it is unlikely that emptying of the stomach will clear more than half of the ingested substance. For this reason, administration of **activated charcoal**, which will absorb most ingested toxins quite efficiently, particularly in the first hour after ingestion, is a mainstay of therapy.

In the present patient, several prescription drugs may have increased morbidity; hypotension and depressed consciousness were probably caused by his cardiac and psychotropic medications. The pine oil–containing household cleaner that he apparently ingested has few specific effects, though a recent series from England suggests that patients ingesting pine oil–containing preparations are at somewhat higher risk of aspiration than those swallowing other substances. The patient was intubated and received gastric lavage via an orogastric tube followed by activated charcoal. He recovered fully, was rapidly removed from the ventilator, and was sent for psychiatric assessment.

Clinical Pearls

1. Attention to the ABCs (airway, breathing, and circulation) remains the cornerstone of therapy for the overdosed or poisoned patient.

2. The most effective means of removing any unabsorbed toxin remaining in the stomach is instillation of activated charcoal. Induction of emesis with ipecac should rarely be performed in adults.

3. Airway protection to prevent aspiration is critical in the poisoned patient with lethargy or loss of consciousness; this may require intubation to allow safe placement of an orogastric tube for lavage or charcoal administration.

REFERENCES

1. Chan TY, Critchley JA, Lau JT. The risk of aspiration in Dettol poisoning: A retrospective study. Hum Exp Toxicol 1995;14:190–191.
2. Pond SM, Lewis-Driver DJ, Williams GM, et al. Gastric emptying in the acute overdose: A prospective randomized controlled trial. Med J Austral 1995;163:345–349.
3. Olson KR. Is gut emptying all washed up? Am J Emerg Med 1990;8:560–561.

PATIENT 10

An 82-year-old woman with shortness of breath and cyanosis

An 82-year-old woman was brought to the emergency department from a nursing home with shortness of breath and cyanosis. Her past medical history included chronic obstructive pulmonary disease (COPD), hypertension, bronchiectasis, and Alzheimer's disease. Medications included albuterol, theophylline, prednisone, and haloperidol.

Physical Examination: Temperature 98°; pulse 100; respirations 28 and shallow; blood pressure 90/56. Chest: bibasilar rales. Neurologic: responsive to verbal stimuli.

Laboratory Findings: WBC 8760/µl, Hct 24.7%, platelets 365,000/µl. Albumin 2.1 g/dl. ABG (100% O_2 non-rebreathing mask): pH 7.54, pCO_2 51 mmHg, pO_2 47 mmHg, HCO_3^- 44 mEq/L, BE 19.3, SaO_2 87%. Sputum Gram stain: gram-negative rods. Chest radiograph (see below): infiltrate to the left upper, left lower, and right lower lobes.

Questions: What are the likely causes of the patient's respiratory failure? What should be the empiric approach to diagnosis and treatment?

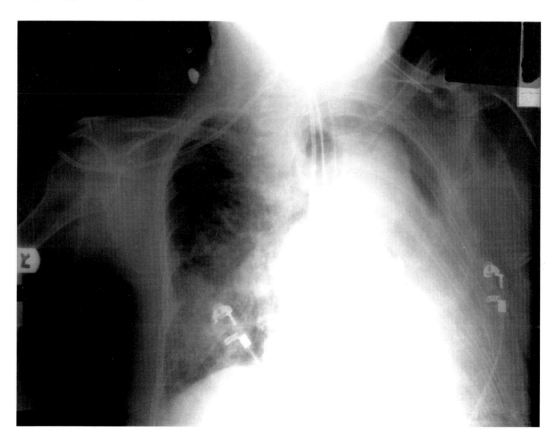

Diagnosis: *Haemophilus influenzae* pneumonia in a patient with underlying COPD.

Discussion: Pneumonia remains a significant cause of morbidity and mortality in the United States. Despite a multitude of new antibiotic agents which have been developed in the past several years, it remains the sixth leading cause of death and the leading cause of death due to infection. It is helpful to classify cases of pneumonia into either community-acquired or hospital-acquired (nosocomial), as etiology and treatment are affected by the setting in which the pneumonia occurs. For example, pneumonia caused by *S. aureus* or gram-negative rods such as *Pseudomonas aeruginosa* often occurs in patients who have been hospitalized, usually in an intensive care unit. These pathogens often affect outpatients with cystic fibrosis, AIDs, intravenous drug use, or other serious conditions.

Several clinical features increase the chance for a poor outcome in patients with community-acquired pneumonia (CAP) and should alert caregivers to the possibility of rapid deterioration in a patient's course. These risk factors include age over 65 years, underlying pulmonary disease (particularly COPD), diabetes mellitus, chronic renal insufficiency, underlying congestive heart failure, chronic liver disease, altered mental status, aspiration, chronic alcohol abuse, and malnutrition. Clinical findings associated with increased morbidity include a respiratory rate greater than 30/minute, hypotension, and temperature greater than 101°. Additionally, laboratory findings of WBC count < 4,000 or > 30,000/μl; PaO_2 < 60 mmHg or $PaCO_2$ > 50 mmHg on room air, a need for mechanical ventilation; multi-lobar involvement on chest radiograph; and the presence of renal insufficiency or other organ dysfunction also define a subset of patients with severe CAP at high risk of dying. The patient in this case clearly met several of these criteria.

Treatment of CAP is usually empiric and is determined by the prevailing organisms in the community and the characteristics of the patient which might predispose to infection with particular organisms. Recently, organizations such as the American Thoracic Society have de-emphasized extensive diagnostic evaluations unlikely to provide specific or reliable information regarding the etiologic agent of the pneumonia; consequently, there is less reliance on sputum Gram stain and culture. A properly performed Gram stain of an adequate specimen, however, can be of value to broaden the differential diagnosis (rarely, to narrow the antibiotic spectrum). Some advocate bronchoscopy with either quantitative bronchoalveolar lavage fluid culture or culture of material obtained with a protected specimen brush. However, there is little consensus on bronchoscopy, and it is not routinely employed in most centers. Blood cultures are worthwhile since an agent recovered from the blood of a CAP patient probably is the cause of the pneumonia.

Several studies of the etiology of severe CAP (as defined by the above criteria) indicate that the organisms commonly responsible for the syndrome include *Streptococcus pneumoniae, Haemophilus influenzae, Klebsiella pneumoniae,* and *Legionella pneumophila.* For this reason, most guidelines for initial or empiric treatment of severe CAP recommend using a macrolide (to cover *Legionella* spp.) with either an antipseudomonal, third generation cephalosporin, or another antipseudomonal such as a quinolone.

The patient in this case was treated with intravenous erythromycin and ceftazidime. A sputum culture grew *H. influenzae.* Despite aggressive therapy, she died 6 days following admission.

Clinical Pearls

1. Several clinical and laboratory findings are useful in determining which patients with community-acquired pneumonia (CAP) are at high risk for severe complications or death.

2. The etiologic spectrum of CAP requiring admission to the intensive care unit differs from CAP that can be treated outpatient, and includes gram-negative organisms as well as *Legionella pneumophila.*

3. Extensive diagnostic testing is often fruitless in cases of CAP. Rather, therapy should be based on the likely pathogens fitting the clinical and demographic features of the patient.

REFERENCES

1. American Thoracic Society. Guidelines for the initial management of adults with community-acquired pneumonia: Diagnosis, assessment of severity, and initial antimicrobial therapy. Am Rev Respir Dis 1993;148:1418–1426.
2. Rello J, Quintana E, Ausina V. A three-year study of severe community-acquired pneumonia with emphasis on outcome. Chest 1993;103:232–235.
3. Jimenez P, Saldias F, Meneses M, et al. Diagnostic fiberoptic bronchoscopy in patients with community-acquired pneumonia. Comparison between bronchoalveolar lavage and telescoping plugged catheter cultures. Chest 1993;103:1023–1027.

PATIENT 11

A 24-year-old African-American man with fever, shortness of breath, and generalized body ache

A 24-year-old African-American man was brought to the emergency department with fever, vomiting, and generalized body pain that was more pronounced in the back, knees, and head. He reported shortness of breath of 3 days' duration and previous multiple episodes of bone pain.

Physical Examination: Temperature 102.9°; pulse 112; respirations 24; blood pressure 125/65, weight 53 kg, height 69 in. Chest: decreased breath sounds over the right upper lung fields. Extremities: bilateral ulcers over the lower region of the legs. Neurologic: alert and oriented, no focal findings.

Laboratory Findings: WBC 33,000/µl, Hct 17.5%, platelets 487,000/µl. MCV 103.7 Fl, MCH 35.3 pg, Na^+ 129 mEq/L, K^+ 4.5 mEq/L, CL^- 89 mEq/L, HCO_3^- 14 mEq/L. ABG (FiO_2 0.50, by face mask): pH 7.33, pCO_2 26 mmHg, pO_2 80 mmHg, SaO_2 95%. Chest radiograph (see below): right upper lobe and lingular infiltrates.

Question: What is the diagnosis?

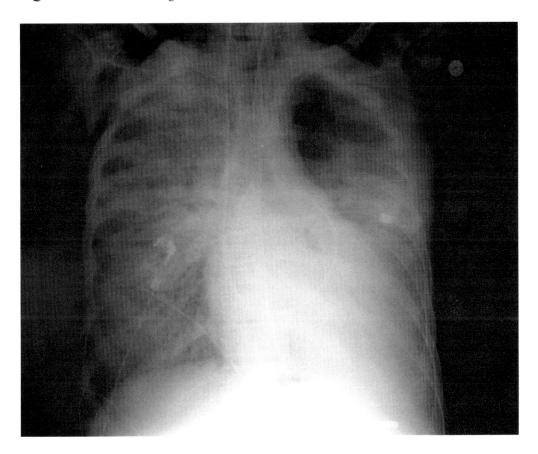

Diagnosis: Sickle cell anemia with pneumonia and acute chest syndrome.

Discussion: Sickle cell anemia is a common genetic disorder in the United States. The disease is inherited in an autosomal recessive fashion, and as many as 8–10% of African-Americans are carriers of the gene for hemoglobin S. Carriers are not clinically affected, but those with two copies of the abnormal gene are subject to the hemolysis and repeated episodes of painful vascular occlusive crises which are the hallmark of this debilitating disease.

Pulmonary complications of sickle cell anemia are common and fall into two major categories: (infectious and noninfectious. Infections are common in patients with the disease. Repeated vascular occlusive events lead to functional asplenism in many sickle cell patients, leaving them vulnerable to infection by encapsulated organisms, chief among them *Streptococcus pneumoniae*. For this reason, all patients with sickle cell anemia receive the pneumococcal vaccine, preferably before the spleen has become completely nonfunctional. Children with the disease also receive prophylactic treatment with penicillin. These strategies have reduced morbidity from pneumococcal infection, and organisms such as *Hemophilus influenzae* now assume a prominent role in infectious complications of sickle cell disease.

Noninfectious pulmonary complications of sickle cell disease are generally related to vascular occlusion. In situ vascular occlusion, pulmonary embolism, and fat embolism from infarcted bone can all cause clinical illness in these patients, with chest pain, tachypnea, infiltrates and consolidation seen on chest radiograph, and severe hypoxemia resulting. Acute respiratory distress syndrome has been noted to develop as a result of these vascular crises.

Obviously, the syndromes caused by bacterial pneumonia and vascular occlusion can be extremely difficult to distinguish on clinical grounds. For this reason, patients with sickle cell anemia who present with fever, chest pain, hypoxemia, and infiltrates seen on chest radiograph are said to have **"acute chest syndrome."** Though carefully performed studies in patients with acute chest syndrome indicate that infection is usually not present in those older than 5 years, it is impossible to exclude infection on clinical grounds, and essentially all patients presenting with the syndrome must receive antibiotics in addition to fluids, oxygen, and analgesia.

Prevention of clinical deterioration in acute chest syndrome may be aided by early use of incentive spirometry in patients admitted with chest pain but no infiltrates on chest radiograph. A recent, controlled trial of this technique indicated that patients performing 10 maximal inspirations every two hours while awake developed significant pulmonary complications (manifested by radiographic abnormalities and hypoxia) on only 1 of 19 occasions, whereas complications occurred on 8 of 19 occasions when the technique was not used.

For patients who develop refractory hypoxemia and extensive pulmonary infiltrates, partial exchange transfusion may play a role as a therapeutic maneuver, with the goal of increasing the hemoglobin A concentration to 50–60% of the total. There is no evidence, however, that aggressive transfusion practices prevent the development of acute chest syndrome.

The patient in this case required mechanical ventilation for worsening hypoxia and pulmonary infiltrates. Despite therapy with fluids, antibiotics, oxygen, and analgesia, he died on the seventh hospital day.

Clinical Pearls

1. Pulmonary complications are common in patients with sickle cell anemia, including infection, pulmonary infarction, pulmonary embolism, and fat embolism. Pneumococcal vaccine should be given to all sickle cell patients early in life to reduce infectious complications.

2. Patients with acute chest syndrome (fever, chest pain, hypoxemia, and pulmonary infiltrates) should be treated with antibiotics routinely, as infection cannot be excluded on clinical grounds.

3. Patients admitted with chest or upper back pain may benefit from early and frequent use of incentive spirometry.

REFERENCES
1. Godeau B, Schaeffer A, Bachir D, et al. Bronchoalveolar lavage in adult sickle cell patients with acute chest syndrome: Value for diagnostic assessment of fat embolism. Am J Respir Crit Care Med 1996:153:1691–1696.
2. Bellet PS, Kalinyak KA, Shukla R, et al. Incentive spirometry to prevent acute pulmonary complications in sickle cell diseases. N Engl J Med 1995;333:699–703.
3. Vichinsky EP, Haberkern CM, Neumayr L, et al. A comparison of conservative and aggressive transfusion regimens in the perioperative management of sickle cell disease. The Preoperative Transfusion in Sickle Cell Disease Study Group. N Engl J Med 1995:333:206–213.
4. Weil JV, Castro O, Malik AB, et al. National Heart, Lung, and Blood Institute Workshop Summary. Pathogenesis of lung disease in sickle hemoglobinopathies. Am Rev Respir Dis 1993;148:249–256.

PATIENT 12

A 61-year-old man with exertional dyspnea, pedal edema, two-pillow orthopnea, and increased sputum production

A 61-year-old obese man presented to his physician's office complaining of difficulty sleeping, somnolence, and headaches upon awakening. He had a 28-pack-year smoking history and previously had been diagnosed with chronic obstructive pulmonary disease (COPD). Current medications included theophylline, prednisone, and albuterol and beclomethasone metered-dose inhalers. His wife claimed that he had periods of "not breathing" and loud snoring while asleep. The patient admitted that he has fallen asleep while driving.

Physical Examination: Temperature 98.6°; pulse 75; respirations 20; blood pressure 130/80. Chest: Bilateral expiratory wheezing with rhonchi. Extremities: ++ pedal edema.

Laboratory Findings: SpO_2 (room air) 94%. Prior PFTs: see table.

Pulmonary Function Tests

	Pre Bronchodilator		Post Bronchodilator	
	Actual	% Predicted	Actual	% Predicted
FVC	1.93 L	41	2.78 L	59
FEV_1	0.95 L	25.8	1.50 L	40.8
FEV_3	1.51 L	34.8	2.32 L	53.4
FEV_1/FVC	49.2%	62.9	54.0%	69.1
FEV_3/FVC	78.5%	85	83.4%	90.4
PEF	2.51 L/S	29.2	3.68 L/S	42.8
FEF_{25-75}	0.41 L/S	11.5	0.72 L/S	20.3

L/S = liters per second.

Questions: What is the most likely diagnosis for this patient? What is an appropriate respiratory therapy intervention based upon the clinical data?

Diagnosis: Obstructive sleep apnea in a patient with COPD.

Discussion: It is increasingly recognized that obstructive sleep apnea syndrome (OSAS) is more common than had previously been appreciated. Early estimates put the prevalence at 0.3–1.0% of the middle-aged population, but more recent studies indicate a prevalence substantially higher. Using a definition of the syndrome as an apnea-hypopnea index (AHI) > 5, one study determined the prevalence in middle-aged women to be 9%, and in men to be 24%. This would make OSAS as common as asthma. Though it has been difficult to separate the contribution of OSAS to overall mortality from the contributions of other conditions that often accompany it (such as hypertension, obesity, and cardiovascular disease), fatal automobile and industrial accidents have been attributed to patients with undiagnosed sleep apnea falling asleep while performing these activities. Nevertheless, OSAS is still an under-recognized disorder.

Sleep apnea is defined as an intermittent cessation of airflow at the nose and mouth during sleep. The complete syndrome is characterized by repetitive episodes of **upper airway obstruction** during sleep, usually associated with a reduction in arterial blood oxygen saturation; **loud snoring** during sleep; and **daytime hypersomnolence** resulting from the interrupted, fragmented sleep caused by the apneic episodes. These last two characteristics may be considered cardinal symptoms. The immediate factor leading to collapse of the upper airway is still a matter of some debate, though most believe that the collapse results from either an abnormal loss of upper airway tone during sleep or an inability to normally increase tone during REM sleep, which is when apneas occur.

Diagnosis of OSAS rests on demonstration of recurrent sleep apneas, formally established by polysomnography, in which airflow at the nose and arterial oxygen saturation are measured in a subject during sleep. However, loud, disruptive snoring and apneic periods observed by a spouse or bed partner can be strong predictors of the presence of OSAS. The self-reported symptom of sleepiness alone, in the absence of the other features previously noted or formal sleep latency testing, is a less reliable predictor of the syndrome. Similarly, though most patients with sleep apnea are obese, physical findings such as neck circumference or tonsil size are not useful predictors. Pulmonary function testing and arterial blood gas analysis also are unreliable, as these tests in awake OSAS patients can be normal unless there is a superimposed component of COPD or central apnea.

Once diagnosed, the specific choice of treatment depends on the severity of OSA. Mild to moderate OSA can be effectively managed by weight reduction, though this is difficult to sustain. Severe OSA can be effectively treated with nasal, continuous positive airway pressure (CPAP, or BiPAP), which acts as a pneumatic splint to maintain upper airway patency during REM sleep. This therapy is effective, but patient acceptance of the therapy often wanes over time due to the discomfort sometimes associated with the CPAP apparatus. Uvulopalatopharyngoplasty (UVPP), the removal of the tonsils and adenoids, uvula, distal margin of the soft palate, and any excessive pharyngeal tissue, is reserved for severe cases, and the identification of patients who will benefit most from this procedure is inexact. Tracheostomy is generally curative in OSAS, though this is obviously a somewhat drastic measure.

The present patient underwent a polysomnogram (5 hours, 10 minutes). The index of disordered breathing was 28.56 events with the longest apneic period lasting 2 minutes, 14 seconds. The mean oxygen saturation was 82% with a low of 50%. REM sleep was documented at 20%. He is currently maintained on 12.5/5 cm H_2O BiPAP with 2 L/min of supplemental nocturnal oxygen, and he sleeps comfortably throughout the night.

Clinical Pearls

1. Although OSA may occur at any age, the typical patient is a male aged 30–60 years with a history of snoring, moderate obesity, and excessive daytime sleepiness.

2. BiPAP or CPAP is considered the respiratory care treatment of choice in patients diagnosed with OSA. Titration of this therapy is critical to achieve optimal results.

3. Supplemental nocturnal oxygen therapy should be used only in patients with documented hypoxemia and/or periods of desaturation.

REFERENCES

1. Strohy KP, Redline S. Recognition of obstructive sleep apnea. Am J Respir Crit Care Med 1996;154:279–289.
2. Young T, Palta M, Dempsey J, et al. The occurrence of sleep disordered breathing among middle-aged adults. N Engl J Med 1993;328:1230–1235.
3. Fujita S. Obstructive sleep apnea syndrome: Pathophysiology, upper airway evaluation and surgical treatment. Ear Nose Throat J 1993;72:77.
4. Rodenstein DO. Assessment of uvulopalatopharyngoplasty for the treatment of sleep apnea syndrome. Sleep 1992;15:S56–62.

PATIENT 13

A 51-year-old man with severe shortness of breath and hemoptysis

A 51-year-old man was brought to the emergency department complaining of severe shortness of breath and hemoptysis for the previous 3 days. The patient had been well until 4 months earlier when he had developed cough occasionally productive of blood and was found to have pulmonary tuberculosis. He had responded well to therapy and his initial cough had subsided. Medications included isoniazid, rifampin, ethambutol, famotidine, and vitamin B_6.

Physical Examination: Temperature 99.1°; pulse 100; respirations 24; blood pressure 140/90. Chest crackles over the entire left lung with absent breath sounds on the right. Extremities: clubbing present. Neurologic: alert and oriented.

Laboratory Findings: WBC 13,700/μl, Hct 32%. Albumin 3 g/dl, GGT 122 IU/L, LDH 952 IU/L. ABG (non-breathing mask): pH 7.42, pCO_2 40 mmHg, pO_2 71 mmHg, HCO_3^- 25 mEq/L, SaO_2 94%. Chest radiograph (see below): complete opacification of the right lung. Flexible fiberoptic bronchoscopy revealed a mass in the right main bronchus with a large adherent clot completely obscuring the lumen.

Questions: What is the cause of the patient's sudden dyspnea? What special respiratory care considerations exist for this patient?

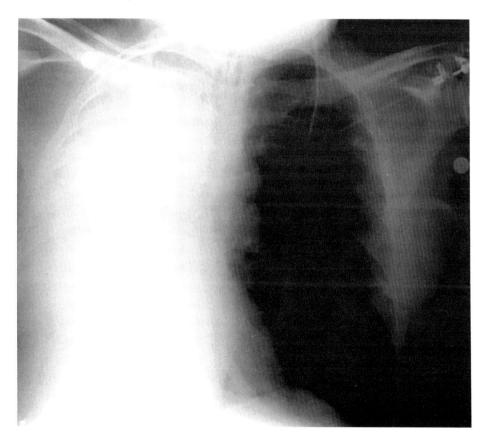

Diagnosis: Obstruction of the right main bronchus due to carcinoma.

Discussion: Sudden dyspnea can have a variety of causes, such as pneumothorax, asthma, and pulmonary embolism, but **airway obstruction** should be a leading consideration when a patient presents with sudden shortness of breath, diminished breath sounds over one hemithorax, and a chest radiograph demonstrating opacification of one lung. Usually, obstruction of the right or left main bronchus results in significant volume loss and a shift of the mediastinal structures toward the opacified lung. A coexisting pleural effusion, such as is often seen in the setting of bronchogenic carcinoma, can balance this shift so that the mediastinal structures remain more or less in the midline. Though aspiration of a foreign body is a common cause of airway obstruction, endobronchial neoplasms, lymphadenopathy, and extraluminal mass lesions compressing the bronchus can also lead to dyspnea.

The severity of dyspnea associated with the obstruction is usually related to the time over which the obstruction developed. Aspiration of a foreign body and bleeding that occludes an airway cause the most severe dyspnea because of sudden ventilation/perfusion imbalance, whereas a slowly growing mass lesion compressing an airway over several weeks causes only minimal symptoms as pulmonary blood flow shifts away from the unventilated lung.

Bronchoscopy is an invasive procedure that allows direct visualization of the tracheobronchial tree, including abnormalities such as tumors and lesions. There are two types of bronchoscopes currently used in clinical practice: the rigid bronchoscope and the fiberoptic bronchoscope. **Rigid bronchoscopy** uses a fixed, wide-bore metal tube that incorporates a lighted lens system. It is most helpful in the removal of foreign bodies and when small biopsy suction channels are inadequate. Some advocate it in cases of massive hemoptysis because of the better suctioning possible with rigid scopes. However, rigid bronchoscopy requires general anesthesia and does not allow inspection much beyond the orifices of the right and left main bronchi.

Flexible bronchoscopy uses fiberoptic illumination to visualize respiratory structures including the segmental and subsegmental bronchi. The distal tip can be flexed easily to angles exceeding 90°. Additionally, biopsy forceps, catheters, and brushes can be passed through the scope to accomplish transbronchial lung biopsy, brushings, or aspiration of secretions for culture or cytologic examination. For mechanically ventilated patients, a variety of adapters ensure the preservation of tidal volume, FiO_2, and positive end-expiratory pressure, so that the fiberoptic bronchoscope can also be used for diagnostic and therapeutic purposes on patients receiving artificial ventilatory support.

Another consideration in a patient with hemoptysis arising from a discrete lesion is protection of the unaffected lung. If in the patient at hand blood began to spill into the left lung, rapid asphyxiation might ensue. Positioning the patient with the bleeding side down may prevent spillage of blood to the unaffected side. (This is contrary to the usual practice of positioning the patient with the abnormal side up, as is done at times for patients with severe unilateral pneumonia in an attempt to improve blood flow to the unaffected lung.) Antitussive medication may reduce the cough. Failing these two measures, insertion of a double-lumen endotracheal tube can occlude the bleeding airway while ventilating the unaffected lung. Insertion of a double-lumen tube must be done by a skilled operator, as its correct function depends on proper placement. Fiberoptic bronchoscopy often aids in positioning.

The present patient was weaned to extubation after thoracentesis and sequential bronchoscopies. He was diagnosed with an inoperable tracheal neoplasm with total occlusion of the right bronchus and moderate constriction of the left bronchus. He is now receiving heliox, chemotherapy, and radiation treatment.

Clinical Pearls

1. Acute bronchial obstruction should be suspected when a patient presents with sudden dyspnea and an opacified hemithorax with shift of the mediastinum toward the side of opacification.

2. Flexible fiberoptic bronchoscopy, because of its ready availability and versatility, is a useful tool for initial inspection in most cases of suspected airway obstruction.

3. The use of double-lumen endotracheal tubes can reduce the chance of contamination of an unaffected lung by a bleeding source.

REFERENCES
1. Kato R, Sawafuji M, Kawamura M, et al. Massive hemoptysis successfully treated by modified bronchoscopic balloon tamponade technique. Chest 1996;109:842–843.
2. Helmers RA, Sanderson DR. Rigid bronchoscopy. The forgotten art. Clin Chest Med 1995;16:393–399.
3. Freitag L. Development of a new balloon catheter for management of hemoptysis with bronchofibrescopes. Chest 1993;103:593.

PATIENT 14

A 57-year-old man with shortness of breath and bilateral wheezing

A 57-year-old man was brought to the emergency department by ambulance complaining of shortness of breath with bilateral wheezing for 1 day. The patient was asymptomatic until 1 week prior when he developed similar but less severe symptoms after walking outside for 5 minutes. Medications included albuterol via metered-dose inhaler.

Physical Examination: Temperature 98.8°; pulse 120; respirations 36; blood pressure 220/86. General: using accessory muscles; in significant respiratory difficulty. Chest: diffuse wheezes with poor air entry. Neurologic: alert and oriented, although extremely anxious.

Laboratory Findings: WBC 14,000/μl, glucose 147 mg/dl. ABG (FiO$_2$ 1.0): pH 7.15, pCO$_2$ 69 mmHg, pO$_2$ 51 mmHg, HCO$_3^-$ 24 mEq/L, SaO$_2$ 75%. Peak flow was unobtainable due to his tachypnea. Chest radiograph (see below): hyperinflation without evidence of infiltrate or congestion.

Questions: What condition most likely explains the patient's clinical presentation? What guidelines should be followed in determining when intubation is indicated in this patient?

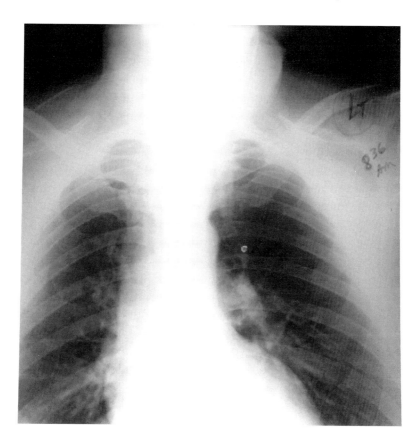

Diagnosis: Acute exacerbation of cold-induced asthma.

Discussion: Asthma is an extremely common respiratory disorder in the United States and other industrialized countries. It is estimated that 12–20 million Americans have asthma, and although most of these patients can be managed quite well with currently available medications, life-threatening episodes of asthma occur not infrequently. Although death from asthma is not common, it is disturbing to note that asthma mortality has been rising in the U.S., particularly in urban areas. It is not clear whether this is because of more severe disease in these areas (perhaps due to pollution or poorly ventilated, older apartment buildings, especially in poor neighborhoods) or because of a lack of access to good medical care. Whatever the cause, a severe asthma attack represents one of the most serious challenges to the pulmonary physician and respiratory therapist.

Asthmas is characterized by *reversible* airways obstruction. Previously, the airways obstruction was believed to be largely due to bronchial smooth muscle contraction, and treatment was mostly aimed at reversing this muscle contraction with bronchodilators such as aminophylline and beta-adrenergic agonists. However, in the past several years, it has become clear that a major component of the airways obstruction in asthma is **inflammation**. There is a large influx of inflammatory cells and cytokines into the airways of asthmatic patients in response to a variety of stimuli, including allergens, infection, cold air, and other substances. With the recognition of the importance of the inflammatory component has come a major emphasis on the use of anti-inflammatory drugs, primarily corticosteroids, as mainstays of asthma treatment. In addition, the role of other pro-inflammatory substances, primarily the arachidonic acid derivatives such as leukotrienes LTB_4, LTC_4, and LTD_4, has led to the development of drugs that can block either the synthesis of these substances (such as the 5-lipoxygenase inhibitors) or their mode of action (leukotriene receptor antagonists). These drugs are expected to reach the market in the near future.

For patients with severe bronchospasm presenting with acute respiratory acidosis, such as the present patient, therapy must be provided immediately and the patient must be closely observed for possible respiratory arrest. Immediate administration of inhaled (usually via nebulizer) **beta-agonists** is the mainstay of therapy. These drugs can be given continuously until the bronchospasm improves. Other agents such as aminophylline and epinephrine probably add to toxicity without providing much benefit as bronchodilators. Magnesium sulfate has not been convincingly demonstrated to be useful in this situation. Corticosteroids, usually in the form of intravenous methylprednisolone, should be given, though the onset of their action will not be immediate. They are, however, helpful in treating the so-called late-phase response with its substantial inflammatory component.

Occasionally, a patient presenting with status asthmaticus does not respond to bronchodilator therapy and requires intubation and institution of mechanical ventilation. Management of intubated asthmatics can be extremely difficult, owing to the high airway pressure and mucus plugging often seen. Neuromuscular blockade and/or general anesthesia may be necessary in order to achieve adequate tidal volume and minute ventilation; deliberate hypoventilation (permissive hypercapnia) may also help to reduce the risk of barotrauma and auto-PEEP.

The present patient was treated with epinephrine, methylprednisolone, aminophylline, aerosolized albuterol, and oxygen. He responded well to this therapy and was discharged 72 hours after admission.

Clinical Pearls

1. In the treatment of status asthmaticus, beta-agonists provide the fastest and most substantial relief of bronchoconstriction. Other bronchodilators such as epinephrine and aminophylline add little to bronchodilation and increase the chance of adverse effects.

2. Steroids should be given to all asthmatic patients in the emergency department who did not respond immediately to a dose of inhaled beta-agonists.

3. Asthmatic patients requiring mechanical ventilation must be managed carefully owing to their high airway pressure and risk of auto-PEEP and barotrauma.

REFERENCES

1. Corbridge TC, Hall JB. The assessment and management of adults with status asthmaticus. Am J Respir Crit Care 1995;151:1296–1316.
2. Bellomo R, McLaughlin P, Tai E, Parkin G. Asthma requiring mechanical ventilation. A low morbidity approach. Chest 1194;105:891–896.
3. Papo MC, Frank J, Thompson AE. A prospective, randomized study of continuous versus intermittent nebulized albuterol for severe status asthmaticus in children. Crit Care Med 1993;21:1479–1486.
4. Miller TP, Greenberger PA, Patterson R. The diagnosis of potentially fatal asthma in hospitalized adults: Patient characteristics and increased severity of asthma. Chest 1992;102:515–518.

PATIENT 15

A 92-year-old woman with respiratory distress immediately after extubation

A 92-year-old woman complained of severe difficulty breathing twenty minutes following extubation. She had been admitted to the hospital 4 days earlier for treatment of pneumonia and congestive heart failure and had required mechanical intubation due to respiratory failure. Past medical history included oxygen-dependent COPD, CHF, and recurrent pneumonias requiring four intubations during the past 3 years.

Physical Examination: Temperature 100.4°; pulse 94; respirations 32 and labored; blood pressure 122/70. Chest: scattered crackles and a high pitched musical sound noted over the trachea. Cardiac: regular rate and rhythm. Neurologic: anxious, nonfocal. Extremities: without cyanosis, clubbing, or edema.

Laboratory Findings: WBC 15,000/µl, Hct 30.6%, platelets 336,000/µl. Na$^+$ 139 mEq/L, K$^+$ 5.1 mEq/L, Cl$^-$ 94 mEq/L, HCO$_3^-$ 24 mEq/L. BUN 58 mg/dl, Cr 1.3 mg/dl. ABG (non-breathing mask): pH 7.62, pCO$_2$ 23 mmHg, pO$_2$ 254 mmHg, SaO$_2$ 99%. Chest radiograph on admission to the ICU (see below): left lower lobe infiltrate.

Question: What is the cause of respiratory distress in this patient?

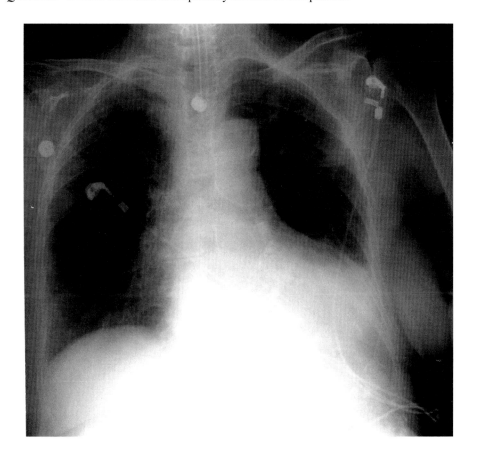

Diagnosis: Subglottic edema post extubation.

Discussion: Respiratory distress immediately following extubation and discontinuation of mechanical intubation can have many causes but, in broad terms, it is usually related either to insufficient resolution of the illness that required ventilatory assistance in the first place or to the development of a new complication related to mechanical ventilation or tracheal intubation. If a patient is observed breathing comfortably on minimal ventilatory support (for example, on a T-piece without assisted breaths) prior to extubation, respiratory distress soon after extubation suggests upper airway disease possibly caused by (and masked during mechanical ventilatory support by) endotracheal intubation. Cases such as these serve as reminders that mechanical ventilation is not always a benign endeavor. Though complications such as ventilator-associated pneumonia and pneumothorax are well recognized, damage to the upper airway from translaryngeal intubation is another potentially serious form of morbidity associated with mechanical ventilation.

Upper airway complications resulting from translaryngeal intubation begin in the paranasal sinuses and extend to the trachea. Sinusitis can be a serious problem in endotracheal intubation, particularly for transnasal approaches, but it is unlikely to present as respiratory distress following extubation. Similarly, oral complications of intubation such as facial cellulitis and lip ulcerations should not cause respiratory difficulty. Pharyngeal complications of intubation include sore throat and dysphagia, which are usually not serious, though persistent dysphagia can result in a cricoid abscess requiring drainage. A potentially more serious pharyngeal complication is loss of the **gag reflex**, which can lead to aspiration—certainly a cause of respiratory distress. For this reason, recently extubated patients should not be fed until the gag reflex has been tested and deemed adequate.

Laryngeal lesions can cause the most serious respiratory distress following removal of the endotracheal tube. Damage to the vocal cords has been documented in a majority of patients following extubation, and in a few instances lesions such as ulcerations prevented cord adduction, predisposing patients to aspiration. More serious laryngeal complications of intubation include edema, laryngospasm, stridor, and vocal cord paralysis, all of which can occur early (in the first week) after extubation. Later complications include glottic and subglottic stenosis with fibrosis, and granuloma formation.

Stridor, the symptom in the patient presented in this case, occurs in 0.1–0.6% of patients following extubation and can have several anatomic correlates. Usually stridor in this setting is caused by vocal cord edema or subglottic swelling and stenosis rather than laryngospasm. Risk factors for the development of stridor include repeated intubation or tracheotomy.

The management of patients with stridor following extubation includes the usual types of supportive care as well as some specific measures to reduce upper airway edema. Typically, racemic epinephrine (2.25%) is used to reduce swelling, though a recent study indicates that the less expensive and more widely available L-epinephrine (1%) is equally effective, with less tachycardia and other cardiovascular effects. Heliox (a mixture of 80% helium and 20% oxygen) may provide less turbulent flow and better oxygenation, but provision is limited by the need for blenders to prepare the mixture, and the therapy cannot be used in patients requiring high inspired-oxygen concentrations. As stridor is an uncommon complication of translaryngeal intubation, prophylactic administration of racemic epinephrine is not warranted. In patients with stridor and multiple intubations, prednisone administered several hours prior to extubation may be helpful.

The patient in this case responded transiently to aerosolized racemic epinephrine but required reintubation 1 hour after extubation. After a 36-hour administration of intravenous steroids, she was successfully extubated and remained so with serial racemic epinephrine treatments over 12 hours.

Clinical Pearls

1. Respiratory distress soon after extubation may suggest an upper airway problem related to translaryngeal intubation if the underlying cause of the patient's respiratory failure has been corrected.

2. Stridor in a recently extubated patient suggests laryngeal edema or subglottic stenosis.

3. L-epinephrine may be as effective as racemic epinephrine for the treatment of laryngeal edema. Prophylactic corticosteroids should be used only in patients with repeated intubations and prior episodes of stridor.

REFERENCES

1. Dalton C. Bilateral vocal cord paralysis following endotracheal intubation. Anesth Intens Care 1995;23:350–351.
2. Nutman J, Brooks LJ, Deakins KM, et al. Racemic versus L-epinephrine aerosol in the treatment of post extubation laryngeal edema: Results from a prospective, randomized, double-blind study. Crit Care Med 1994;22:1591–1594.
3. Sukhani R, Barclay J, Chow J. Paradoxical vocal cord motion: An unusual cause of stridor in the recovery room. Anesthesiology 1993;79:177–180.
4. Golice GL. Resolution of laryngeal injury following translaryngeal intubation. Am Rev Respir Dis 1992;145:361–364.
5. Colice GL, Stukel TA, Dain B. Laryngeal complications of prolonged intubation. Chest 1989;96:877–884.

PATIENT 16

A 56-year-old man with hypertension, persistent headache, and irregular respirations

A 56-year-old man was brought to the emergency department complaining of 4 days of dyspnea, dizziness, and an episode of near fainting. His past medical history included hypertension, cardiomyopathy, non-insulin–dependent diabetes mellitus, and a left-hemispheric stroke three years ago without residual effects. His medications included captopril, nifedipine, hydralazine, and glyburide.

Physical Examination: Temperature 97.3°; pulse 92; respirations 32 and irregular, with a series of deep breaths alternating with a series of shallow ones; blood pressure 220/110. Chest: rhonchi bilaterally. Neurologic: expressive aphasia with right-sided weakness.

Laboratory Findings: Na^+ 138 mEq/L, K^+ 3.7 mEq/L, Cl^- 103 mEq/L, HCO_3^- 24 mEq/L. Glucose 179 mg/dl, BUN 21 mg/dl, Cr 1.2 mg/dl. Chest radiograph (see below): cardiomegaly with pulmonary congestion and reticulonodular densities. ABG (50% oxygen by face mask): pH 7.47, pCO_2 27 mmHg, pO_2 85 mmHg, SaO_2 97%.

Question: What are the type and cause of the abnormal ventilatory pattern described in this patient?

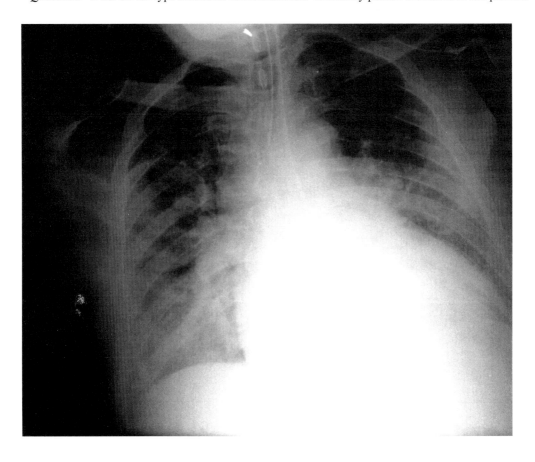

Diagnosis: Cheyne-Stokes respirations in a patient with cerebrovascular disease and congestive heart failure.

Discussion: There are a variety of abnormal respiratory patterns seen in clinical practice, and their correct identification can lead to improved therapy for the **underlying disease state** with which they are associated. Several abnormal patterns are linked to very specific lesions in the nervous system: derangement of automatic respiration is associated with Biot's respirations (a random and disorganized mix of deep and shallow respirations), which also usually are due to medullary disease, and apneustic respirations (a pattern of breathing characterized by sustained inspiratory pauses) are associated with damage in the midpons often caused by basilar artery infarction. One of the most well-recognized and studied of the abnormal respiratory patterns, Cheyne-Stokes respiration, is a ventilatory pattern characterized by oscillations of gradually increasing and then decreasing tidal volumes, separated by relatively brief periods of apnea. Though most commonly associated with central nervous system disease (including diffuse disorders such as metabolic encephalopathies), Cheyne-Stokes respirations often accompany **congestive heart failure**, and this association has been the subject of much investigation in recent years. There is now recognition that a variety of abnormal respiratory patterns are associated with congestive failure.

A recent study of 100 consecutive patients with clinically well-controlled, moderately severe (mean ejection fraction 34%) heart failure found that Cheyne-Stokes breathing was present in 27 subjects, and an additional 43 patients had a variety of other ventilatory pattern disorders, including nonspecific periods of apneas and hypopneas. Patients with Cheyne-Stokes respirations had an average of 24 episodes of oxyhemoglobin desaturations per hour. Predictors of the presence of Cheyne-Stokes respirations included a history of **nocturnal dyspnea** and **atrial fibrillation**. Furthermore, a second study indicated that patients with congestive heart failure and Cheyne-Stokes breathing had significantly more daytime somnolence, as assessed by sleep latency, and significantly less REM sleep than both patients with congestive heart failure without Cheyne-Stokes breathing and healthy controls. It also has been suggested that the presence of Cheyne-Stokes breathing in patients with congestive heart failure is an independent predictor of mortality.

The cause of Cheyne-Stokes respirations in patients with congestive heart failure is unknown, though some experimental work suggests that the breathing pattern may be a manifestation of an abnormal CO_2 response; Cheyne-Stokes breathing is more likely to occur in patients with CHF who manifest hypocapnia during wakefulness. Care obviously includes treatment of the underlying cardiac pathophysiology, but specific measures aimed at the respiratory abnormality may be helpful. The application of simple nocturnal oxygen has been associated with an improvement in exercise capacity (as assessed by an improvement in maximal O_2 uptake during exercise) and briefer duration of Cheyne-Stokes breathing. Several studies have indicated that nasal continuous-positive airway pressure (CPAP) also is effective in treating this abnormal breathing pattern as well as improving cardiac function, perhaps by reducing peripheral catecholamine concentrations. Symptomatic improvement also has been noted following administration of benzodiazepines.

The present patient was treated with oxygen, diuretics, and angiotensin-converting enzyme inhibitors, with improvement in congestive heart failure and alleviation of Cheyne-Stokes breathing pattern.

Clinical Pearls

1. Though commonly associated with a variety of primary central nervous system disorders, Cheyne-Stokes respirations are increasingly recognized as a part of the syndrome of congestive heart failure.

2. Cheyne-Stokes breathing in patients with CHF is associated with excessive daytime sleepiness, reduced duration of REM sleep, and increased mortality.

3. After correction of the cardiac disorder to the extent possible, treatment of Cheyne-Stokes breathing in patients with CHF can include nocturnal oxygen or nasal CPAP to improve respiratory symptoms as well as overall cardiac function.

REFERENCES

1. Andreas S, Clemens S, Sandholzer H, et al. Improvement of exercise capacity with treatment of Cheyne-Stokes respiration in patients with congestive heart failure. J Am Coll Cardiol 1996;27:1486–1490.
2. Granton JT, Naughton MT, Benard DC, et al. CPAP improves inspiratory muscle strength in patients with heart failure and central sleep apnea. Am J Respir Crit Care Med 1996;153:277–282.
3. Hanly PJ, Zuberi-Khokhar NS. Increased mortality associated with Cheyne-Stokes respiration in patients with congestive heart failure. Am J Respir Crit Care Med 1996;153:272–276.
4. Naughton MT, Benard DC, Liu PP, et al. Effects of nasal CPAP on sympathetic activity in patients with heart failure and central sleep apnea. Am J Respir Crit Care Med 1995;152:473–479.
5. Blackshear JL, Kaplna J, Thopson RC, et al. Nocturnal dyspnea and atrial fibrillation predict Cheyne-Stokes respirations in patients with congestive heart failure. Arch Intern Med 1995;155:1297–1302.

PATIENT 17

A 75-year-old woman with sudden onset of dyspnea

A 75-year-old woman with a history of CHF, chronic renal insufficiency, peptic ulcer disease, and a previous episode of upper gastrointestinal bleeding was brought to the emergency department with sudden onset of dyspnea 2 hours prior.

Physical Examination: Temperature 100.2°; pulse 136; respirations 38; blood pressure 103/68. Chest: fine bilateral basal rales without wheezing. Cardiac: tachycardic. Abdomen: soft, nontender, without masses or organomegaly; stool negative for occult blood. Extremities: +++ pedal edema, no cords palpable, negative Homan's sign. Neurologic: alert and oriented.

Laboratory Findings: BUN 32 mg/dl, Cr 3.5 mg/dl. PT 13.4 sec, PTT 23.6 sec. ABG (100% O_2 via facemask): pH 7.33, pCO_2 57 mmHg, pO_2 41 mmHg, HCO_3^- 27 mEq/L, SaO_2 71%. Chest radiograph (see below): bilateral pleural effusions.

Questions: What is the most likely diagnosis in this patient? What are the general diagnostic tests used in the evaluation of this event?

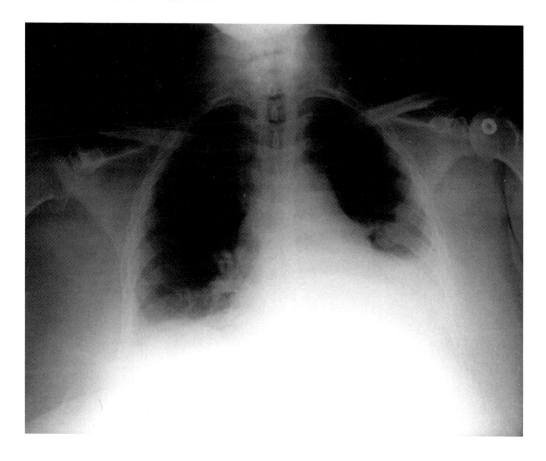

Diagnosis: Pulmonary embolism.

Discussion: Pulmonary embolism (PE) is an extremely common disorder, with roughly 500,000 cases occurring annually in the United States. Most authorities believe that this entity is underdiagnosed, suggesting that a true estimate of morbidity and mortality related to PE is unavailable. It has been pointed out in recent years that PE is actually a symptom of the underlying disease of **deep venous thrombosis** (DVT) and that understanding and preventing the predisposing states for DVT may lead to fewer cases of PE and better outcomes overall. Predisposing conditions to DVT include surgery, obesity, lower extremity trauma, and prolonged immobilization. Risks of DVT associated with surgery are related both to the duration of general anesthesia and to the type of surgery being performed, with the highest risk associated with orthopedic procedures such as total hip and knee arthroplasty. Also recent is an increasing appreciation that acquired and congenital hypercoagulable states, such as those related to malignancy or to protein C deficiency, protein S deficiency, and factor V Leiden deficiency (resulting in resistance to activated protein C), occur in a significant proportion of the population.

Prevention of DVT is the best way to limit morbidity from PE. However, despite prophylactic therapy, substantial numbers of patients present with suspected PE; therefore, a clear approach to diagnosis is essential. The initial step is usually a **ventilation/perfusion (V/Q) scan**, and it is important to properly interpret the information provided by this test. The most helpful data regarding use and interpretation of V/Q scanning was provided by the Prospective Investigation of Pulmonary Embolism Diagnosis (PIOPED) study, which compared V/Q results to pulmonary angiography.

The PIOPED found that although a high-probability V/Q scan carried an 88% chance of being diagnostic for PE, most patients with PE had either an intermediate- or low-probability scan result. Thus, the important finding was that in patients with a significant clinical suspicion of PE, based on risk factors and presenting complaints, any V/Q result other than high probability (which can be considered diagnostic in that setting) or normal must be followed up with further investigation to exclude the diagnosis of PE. Such follow-up can take one of two basic approaches. Since PE is a symptom of the underlying disease of DVT, and the treatment of the two is the same in most cases, making a diagnosis of DVT can usually serve as a surrogate for definitively demonstrating PE. DVT can be diagnosed with non-invasive tests such as duplex Doppler ultrasound (to demonstrate lack of compressibility of the femoral vein) or impedance plethysmography, though both of these tests may be insensitive in calf or asymptomatic proximal thrombosis. If noninvasive testing of the leg is negative in a patient with suspected PE, pulmonary angiogram is still the most direct (and generally quite safe) way of making a diagnosis.

Once a diagnosis of PE has been established, treatment with **anticoagulants** (heparin followed by coumadin) is the standard approach. Vena cava filters are indicated for patients in whom anticoagulants have failed or are contraindicated. The most difficult decisions regarding therapy are usually those regarding use of thrombolytic agents, such as urokinase, streptokinase, or tissue plasminogen activator. In general, these are reserved for patients with massive PE, as evidenced by a greater than 50% perfusion defect or refractory hypotension. More recently, some investigators have suggested using thrombolytics in any patient with PE who has right ventricular dysfunction on echocardiography, but the utility of this approach remains to be demonstrated.

The present patient underwent a V/Q scan which was read as high probability for pulmonary embolism; ascending contrast venography demonstrated deep vein thrombosis. Because of her history of peptic ulcer disease and prior gastrointestinal bleeding, an inferior vena cava umbrella was inserted to prevent further migration of emboli into the pulmonary circulation.

Clinical Pearls

1. Clinical suspicion of PE in patients at risk remains the cornerstone of diagnosis of this disorder, as signs and symptoms are quite nonspecific.

2. V/Q lung scanning is usually the initial step in the diagnostic algorithm for PE. It is most helpful if results show normal or very low probability (essentially excluding PE as a diagnosis) or high probability (making PE very likely). Intermediate probability scans should always be followed up with studies to more definitively demonstrate the presence or absence of DVT or PE.

3. Though anticoagulation is sufficient therapy for most patients with PE, patients with massive emboli, persistent hemodynamic instability, or evidence of right ventricular dysfunction may benefit from thrombolytic therapy.

REFERENCES

1. Weiss K. Pulmonary thromboembolism: Epidemiology and techniques of nuclear medicine. Sem Thromb Hemost 1996;22: 27–32.
2. Lualdi JC, Goldhaber SZ. Right ventricular dysfunction after pulmonary embolism: Pathophysiologic factors, detection, and therapeutic implications. Am Heart J 1995;130:1276–1282.
3. Goldhaber SZ, Haire WD, Feldstein ML, et al. Alteplase versus heparin in acute pulmonary perfusion. Lancet 1993;341: 507–511.
4. Carson JL, Kelley MA, Duff A. The clinical course of pulmonary embolism. New Engl J Med 1992;326:1240–1245.
5. The PIOPED Investigators. Value of the ventilation/perfusion scan in acute pulmonary embolism: Results of the prospective investigation of pulmonary embolism diagnosis. JAMA 1990;263:2753–2759.

PATIENT 18

**A 49-year-old African-American woman with retrosternal chest pain
and dyspnea**

A 49-year-old African-American woman was brought to the emergency department with retrosternal chest pain and dyspnea. She had noted increasing exertional dyspnea superimposed on a background of occasional paroxysmal nocturnal dyspnea and orthopnea. Her past medical history included hypertension, congestive heart failure, and insulin-resistant diabetes mellitus. Medications include verapamil, metoprolol, glypizide, and captopril.

Physical Examination: Temperature 98.8°; pulse 80; respirations 22; blood pressure 168/88. Chest: equal breath sounds with bilateral scattered rales. Abdomen: no masses or organomegaly. Neurologic: nonfocal. Extremities: trace bilateral pedal edema.

Laboratory Findings: CBC and serum electrolytes: normal. Ca^{++} 10.4 mEq/dl, glucose 182 mg/dl. ABG (room air): pH 7.44, pCO_2 36 mmHg, pO_2 85 mmHg, HCO_3^- 25 mEq/L, SaO_2 97%. Chest radiograph (see below): bilateral hilar lymphadenopathy.

Questions: What is the most likely cause of this patient's abnormal chest x-ray? Which diagnostic evaluation is indicated?

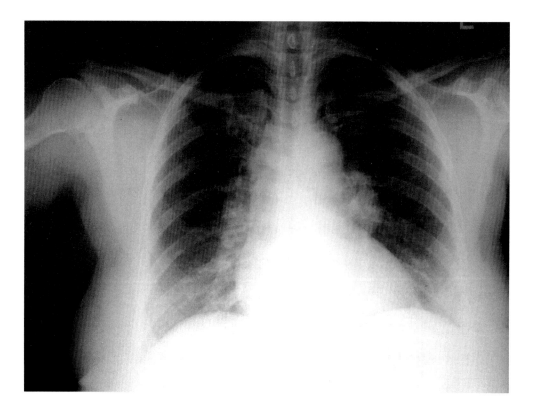

Diagnosis: Pulmonary sarcoidosis.

Discussion: Sarcoidosis is a multisystem, granulomatous disorder of unknown etiology that principally affects the lungs, skin, liver, and lymph nodes, though any organ system may be involved. The diagnosis rests on two key elements: the demonstration of typical, sarcoidal, non-necrotizing granulomas and the exclusion of other known causes of granulomatous inflammation.

Sarcoidosis is a common disease, though in the United States it is unequally distributed among racial and ethnic groups. Its incidence in Caucasians is 5/100,000; in African-Americans 40/100,000. Around the world, sarcoid occurs most commonly in northern Europe and Scandinavia; in Sweden, incidence is 60/1000, and many think that the true incidence is ten-fold higher than that, owing to the large number of asymptomatic individuals. Etiology is unknown, but several features of the disease suggest that sarcoid results from inhalation of an antigenic substance that is processed by antigen-presenting cells, such as alveolar macrophages, which in turn recruit the large number of T-helper lymphocytes that form the **characteristic granulomas** of this disorder. Attempts to identify the offending antigen have been unsuccessful, and several candidate factors, such as unusual forms of mycobacteria or environmental agents such as pine dust, remain unproven as causes of sarcoid.

Clinical manifestations of sarcoid frequently involve the **lung**, though the symptoms are usually nonspecific, such as exertional dyspnea or cough. Physical findings may include lymphadenopathy or hepatosplenomegaly, but the **skin** is the organ most likely to show abnormalities. Skin findings may include erythema nodosum; lupus pernio; or subcutaneous, nodular lesions. The most characteristic findings in sarcoid, however, are those seen on **chest radiograph**. These usually are classified as: type 0, normal; type I (most common), bilateral hilar adenopathy; type II, adenopathy and pulmonary parenchymal lesions together; type III, interstitial changes alone; and type IV, fibrosis and end-stage lung disease. The differential diagnosis in patients with suspected sarcoid is broad; patients with type I and II radiographs may have lymphoma or tuberculosis, whereas those with type III or IV radiographs may have pulmonary fibrosis or chronic hypersensitivity pneumonitis.

Definitive diagnosis of sarcoid rests on demonstrating characteristic granulomas in a tissue biopsy specimen from any involved site. Yield of transbronchial biopsy in patients with abnormal pulmonary parenchyma on chest radiograph is very high, and 65% of patients with hilar adenopathy alone will have positive transbronchial biopsy results. The Kveim test, in which a purified splenic extract taken from a sarcoid patient is injected subcutaneously and the site biopsied 6 weeks later in hopes of demonstrating granuloma formation, is probably sensitive and specific, but the Kveim reagent is not widely available. Nonspecific tests such as gallium scanning or measurement of angiotensin-converting enzyme levels should play little role in the diagnostic evaluation of these patients.

Institution of therapy for pulmonary sarcoid can sometimes be a difficult clinical decision. Many patients are asymptomatic (particularly those with type I radiographs) with normal pulmonary function tests, others demonstrate spontaneous stabilization or improvement. The challenge then is to identify patients who will deteriorate without **steroid therapy**. Close follow-up with radiographs and pulmonary function tests, which may demonstrate worsening lung volumes and diffusion capacity, is probably the best strategy to guide treatment decisions. When steroids are instituted, most experienced clinicians favor fairly prolonged courses of 6–12 months of treatment.

The present patient underwent a pulmonary function test which revealed a minimally decreased vital capacity and DLCO. A transbronchial biopsy showed non-necrotizing granulomas consistent with sarcoid. She is currently being followed in the outpatient chest clinic without treatment.

Clinical Pearls

1. Sarcoidosis is a common lung disorder, but before making the diagnosis, a large number of other pulmonary diseases must be considered, particularly tuberculosis.

2. In sarcoidosis, transbronchial lung biopsy through a fiberoptic bronchoscope usually demonstrates granulomas in the lung parenchyma, even when the chest radiograph does not reveal interstitial lung disease.

3. Nonspecific tests such as gallium scans or measurement of angiotensin-converting enzyme levels should play a minimal role in diagnosis and treatment decisions. Rather, deterioration of vital capacity, gas exchange, or diffusing capacity is typically an indication for the initiation of steroid therapy.

REFERENCES

1. Gibson GJ, Prescott RJ, Muers MF, et al. British Thoracic Society Sarcoidosis Study: Effects of long term corticosteroid treatment. Thorax 1996;51:238–247.
2. Selroos O. Glucocorticosteroids and pulmonary sarcoidosis. Thorax 1996;51:229–230.
3. Lenique F, Brauner MW, Grenier P, et al. CT assessment of bronchi in sarcoidosis: Endoscopic and pathologic correlations. Radiology 1995;194:419–423.
4. Hunninghake GW, Gilbert S, Pueringer R, et al. Outcome of the treatment for sarcoidosis. Am J Respir Crit Care Med 1994;149:893–898.
5. Sharma OP. Pulmonary sarcoidosis and corticosteroids. Amer Rev Respir Dis 1993;147:1598–1600.

PATIENT 19

A 45-year-old man with difficulty breathing, left-side weakness, dysarthria, and severe headache

A 45-year-old man with a history of hypertension was brought to the emergency department complaining of difficulty breathing, left-sided weakness, slurred speech, and severe headache for the prior 4 days.

Physical Examination: Temperature 97.8°; pulse 84; respirations 28 and labored; blood pressure 220/150. Chest: scattered rhonchi. Cardiac: regular rate and rhythm, without murmurs, gallops, or rubs. Abdomen: soft, nontender, without masses or organomegaly. Neurologic: lethargic, slight right pupillary dilatation, gag reflex diminished, slurred speech, marked motor weakness in left upper and lower extremities.

Laboratory Findings: ABG (room air): pH 7.56, pCO_2 26 mmHg, pO_2 105 mmHg, HCO_3^- 22 mEq/L, SaO_2 98%. Chest radiograph (see below): cardiomegaly.

Hospital Course: Upon initial admission, oxygen therapy was continued via non-rebreathing mask and intravenous access was established. While attempting to control systemic blood pressure with nitroprusside and enalapril, the patient's mental status deteriorated. Intubation was performed to control and protect the airway. A CT scan demonstrated intracerebral hemorrhage.

Question: What are the respiratory considerations in the management of this patient, particularly with regard to prevention of nosocomial pneumonia?

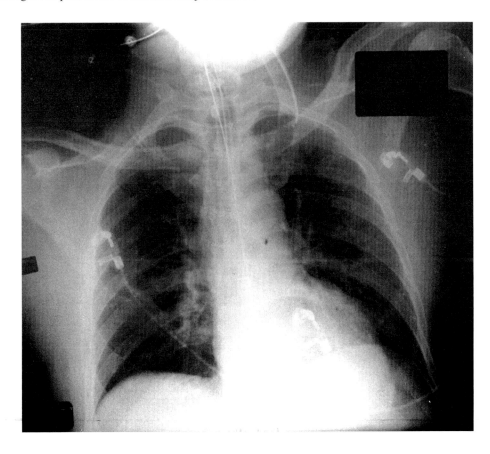

Diagnosis: Hypertensive intracerebral hemorrhage.

Discussion: Morbidity and mortality are related not only to the underlying disease for which the patient is admitted to the intensive care unit, but also to complications that may develop as a result of the invasive procedures commonly performed. Chief among the serious iatrogenic or nosocomial complications occurring in the ICU is **nosocomial, or ventilator-associated, pneumonia**. Nosocomial pneumonia complicates 0.6–1% of hospital admissions in the United States, and the risk of this illness rises dramatically in patients receiving mechanical ventilation, with some studies suggesting as much as a 20-fold increase in incidence. The seriousness of ventilator-associated pneumonia (VAP) is underscored by the bacteriology of the infection. Difficult to treat and virulent pathogens such as *Staphylococcus aureus* and gram negative bacteria such as *Pseudomonas aeruginosa, Serratia marcescens, Enterobacter* spp., and *Acinetobacter* spp. are common causes of pneumonia in this setting.

The development of VAP is related to a variety of factors. Patients with head injury or depressed levels of consciousness, such as the patient presented in this case, often have diminished gag reflexes and are at increased risk of **aspiration** of gastric contents. Endotracheal intubation, often performed with the intention of protecting the airway, does not prevent this complication absolutely—several studies have indicated that it is possible to demonstrate aspiration even around a properly inflated endotracheal tube cuff. The use of nasogastric tubes for enteral feeding may accelerate the risk. Aspiration of oropharyngeal material may be of more concern than aspiration of gastric contents because the former can be colonized with **bacteria** from the hands of health care personnel, including physicians, nurses, and respiratory therapists. Such colonization occurs because of the frequent manipulation of the endotracheal tube, for suctioning and repositioning, and the ventilator tubing and circuitry, for routine changes and the administration of medications via nebulizers.

Reducing the risk of VAP includes treatment of the underlying disorder for which the patient required intubation, thereby minimizing the time the patient spends on the ventilator; appropriate and judicious use of antibiotics to reduce the risk of infection with resistant organisms; and elevation of the patient's head to at least 30°. More complicated techniques, such as selective decontamination of the digestive tract with antibiotic pastes and prophylactic antibiotics, remain controversial and cannot be routinely recommended. Good infection control procedures, such as frequent hand washing and use of gloves and gowns where appropriate, also reduces VAP incidence.

Specific attention to the respiratory care equipment is also of great importance in reducing the risk of nosocomial pneumonia. Recently, it has been convincingly demonstrated that ventilator circuitry only needs to be changed every 48 hours or so; this relatively infrequent manipulation reduces the chance of VAP. Proper removal of the condensation that forms in the tubing, proper disinfection of tubing and nebulizers, careful attention not to transfer equipment between patients, maintenance of humidifiers, and careful handling of in-line medication nebulizers also reduce nosocomial infections.

The present patient underwent a head CT scan which revealed acute hemorrhage with adjacent edema deep in the right fronto-temporal region and right basal ganglia with compression of the right lateral ventricle. With appropriate treatment, the initial symptoms resolved and he suffered no residual deficits. He was weaned from the ventilator quickly and discharged from the hospital on the eleventh day.

Clinical Pearls

1. Nosocomial pneumonia complicates a substantial number of hospital admissions and is a significant cause of morbidity in intubated patients.

2. Prevention of nosocomial pneumonia requires attention to the underlying disorder, infection control procedures, and careful handling of respiratory therapy equipment. Measures such as selective decontamination of the digestive tract are not routinely indicated.

3. Ventilatory circuitry only needs to be changed every 48 hours or so; more frequent manipulation is unnecessary.

REFERENCES

1. Papazian L, Bregeon F, Thirion X, et al. Effect of ventilator-associated pneumonia on mortality and morbidity. Am J Respir Crit Care Med 1996;154:91–97.
2. Rello J, Sonora R, Jubert P, et al. Pneumonia in intubated patients: Role of respiratory airway care. Am J Respir Crit Care Med 1996;154:111–115.
3. Dreyfuss D, Djedaini K, Gros I, et al. Mechanical ventilation with heated humidifiers or heat and moisture exchangers: Effects on patient colonization and incidence of nosocomial pneumonia. Am J Respir Crit Care Med 1995;151:986–992.
4. Estes RJ, Meduri GU. The pathogenesis of ventilator-associated pneumonia: I. Mechanisms of bacterial transcolonization and airway inoculation. Intens Care Med 1995;21:365–383.
5. Duncan RA, Steger KA, Craven DE. Selective decontamination of the digestive tract: Risks outweigh benefits for intensive care unit patients. Semin Respir Infect 1993;8:308–324.
6. George DL. Epidemiology of nosocomial ventilator-associated pneumonia. Infect Control Hosp Epidemiol 1993;14:163–169.

PATIENT 20

A 24-week gestational age, 500-gram infant girl with severe respiratory distress

A 24-week gestational age, 500-gram infant girl was born to a 43-year-old multiparous woman with a history of three spontaneous abortions within the previous 5 years. The mother was transferred to the labor and delivery department after premature rupture of amniotic membranes. Vaginal delivery was performed with an uncomplicated vertex presentation.

Physical Examination: Temperature 94.6°; pulse 157; respirations 59 with nasal flaring and grunting; blood pressure 50/29. Chest: bilateral air entry with inspiratory crackles, with use of accessory muscles. Cardiac: tachycardic. Abdomen: bowel sounds noted. Apgar scores: 5,6. Ballard score: 0.

Laboratory Findings: WBC 23,000/μl, Hct 43%. NA^+ 134 mEq/L, K^+ 4.4 mEq/L, Cl^- 100 mEq/L. Glucose 82 mg/dl, BUN 29 mg/dl, Cr 1.4 mg/dl. Chest radiograph: see below left. Echocardiogram: see below right.

Questions: What is the etiology of the patient's hypoxemia and cyanosis? Which general approaches are used in the management of this patient?

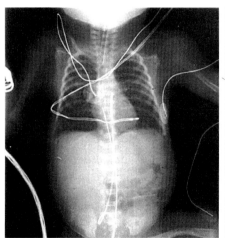 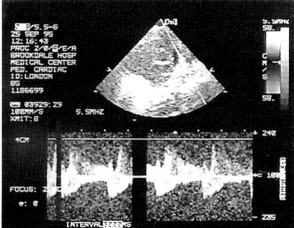

Diagnosis: Patent ductus arteriosus.

Discussion: The differential diagnosis of respiratory disease in a newborn comprises a variety of disorders, and the likely causes vary somewhat with the gestational age at birth. In general, respiratory distress can be separated into more and less common conditions. The most common conditions include transient tachypnea of the newborn (a diagnosis of exclusion), sepsis, aspiration of meconium or amniotic fluid, and metabolic alterations such as hypo- or hyperglycemia or hypo- or hyperthermia. Less common causes of respiratory distress in newborns include congenital infections and congenital heart disease, including the anomalies associated with right-to-left shunting such as tetralogy of Fallot, transposition of the great vessels, total anomalous pulmonary venous return, hypoplastic left heart, Ebstein's anomaly, and truncus arteriosus. Another set of disorders should be included in the differential diagnosis when a **preterm infant** is born with respiratory distress—namely, infant respiratory distress syndrome (hyaline membrane disease), caused by lack of mature surfactant production, and persistence of fetal circulation, which tends to manifest as a patent ductus arteriosus (PDA). During normal fetal development, the ductus arteriosus exists to provide a right-to-left shunt so that maternally-oxygenated blood can pass directly into the left-sided circulation without traversing the fetal lungs. In full-term infants, the ductus generally closes in the first 10–15 hours of life, and only about 8 of 1000 live births are complicated by PDA. However, in preterm infants, the incidence rises dramatically, with PDA occurring in 30–40% of infants weighing less than 1750 grams at birth.

The persistence of PDA results in a left-to-right shunt, pulmonary edema, and left ventricular failure. The left-to-right shunt may be less apparent if there is accompanying hyaline membrane disease, as the resulting increased pulmonary resistance tends to minimize shunting.

Infants with physiologically significant PDA present with respiratory distress, a rhonchorous chest, and a variety of cardiac murmurs. In full-term infants, the characteristic continuous "machinery hum" can suggest the diagnosis, but in preterm newborns, the murmur is more likely to be a rough or "rocky" systolic sound. Chest radiograph and electrocardiogram are unlikely to specifically point to the diagnosis, but **echocardiography** can demonstrate the defect quite readily.

Medical therapy of PDA is the initial approach to treatment. The trigger for a ductus arteriosus to close during normal development is a sudden drop in prostaglandin levels at birth. In the preterm infant, administration of **indomethacin**, which blocks prostaglandin synthesis, can be effective in hastening closure and reducing left-to-right shunt. Recently, a study of prophylactic indomethacin therapy given within 24 hours of birth to infants weighing 600–1250 grams who were being treated with surfactant demonstrated that left-to-right shunting could be diminished by such an approach. Failing a closure with medical therapy, surgical procedures may be considered. These include thoracotomy and division of the arteriosus, or the more recently developed transcatheter closure by placement of a Rashkind umbrella across the patent ductus via a percutaneous technique.

The present patient underwent successful surgical ligation of the ductus arteriosus without complication.

Clinical Pearls

1. Because delayed closure of the ductus arteriosus is associated with respiratory distress syndrome and prematurity, PDA is one of the most common cardiac defects seen in neonatal intensive care units.

2. The definitive diagnosis of PDA is typically made with echocardiography.

3. Medical therapy combined with surgery when needed is associated with a good outcome in the majority of patients.

REFERENCES

1. Couser RJ, Ferrara TB, Wright GB, et al. Prophylactic indomethacin therapy in the first 24 hours of life for the prevention of patent ductus arteriosus in preterm infants treated prophylactically with surfactant in the delivery room. J Pediatr 1996;128:631–637.
2. Weiss H, Cooper B, Brook M, et al. Factors determining reopening of the ductus arteriosus after successful clinical closure with indomethacin. J Pediatr 1995;127:466–471.
3. Archer N. Patent ductus arteriosus in the newborn. Arch Dis Child 1993;69:529–532.
4. Reller MD, Rice MJ, McDonald RW. Review of studies evaluating ductal patency in the premature infant. J Pediatr 1993;122:S59–S62.
5. Peckman GJ, Miettinen OS, Ellison RC, et al. Clinical course to 1 year of age in premature infants with patent ductus arteriosus: Results of a multicenter randomized trial of indomethacin. J Pediatr 1984;105:285–291.

PATIENT 21

A 61-year-old man with persistent air leak following lung resection

A 61-year-old man who was status post right thoracotomy and right upper lobectomy was noted to have a persistently low exhaled tidal volume while on the ventilator. He had been admitted to the hospital for surgery following an episode of hemoptysis caused by an aspergilloma infecting an old, healed tuberculosis cavity.

Physical Examination: Temperature 97.8°; pulse 88; respirations 16; blood pressure 110/70. Chest: rhonchi bilaterally with decreased breath sounds in the right upper lobe. Cardiac: regular rate and rhythm, without murmurs. Abdomen: soft, nontender, without masses or organomegaly. Neurologic: alert and oriented, nonfocal exam.

Laboratory Findings: WBC 23,700/μl, Hct 29%, platelets 230,000/μl. LDH 1388 IU/L, albumin 2.1 gm/dl. ABG (Siemens Servo 900 C ventilator with the following settings: pressure-controlled ventilation, 35 cm H_2O, f = 20, FiO_2 .50, and 6 cm H_2O of PEEP): pH 7.42, pCO_2 33 mmHg, pO_2 95 mmHg, HCO_3^- 22 mEq/L, SaO_2 98%. Chest radiograph: see below.

Questions: What is the likely reason for the persistently low exhaled tidal volume in this patient? Which ventilatory strategies might be followed to minimize the problem?

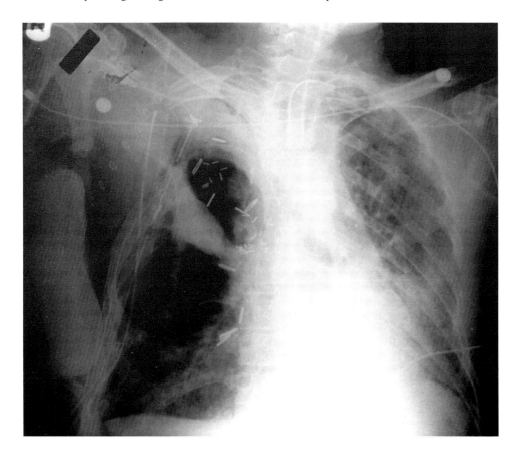

Diagnosis: Bronchopleural fistula following right upper lobe resection.

Discussion: The presence of persistently low exhaled tidal volumes and an air leak noted in the chest tube system is essentially diagnostic of a bronchopleural fistula (BPF). Though bronchopleural fistulas can complicate a variety of pulmonary disorders including necrotizing pneumonias and tuberculosis, such as complication usually develops in one of two settings: **postoperatively** following resectional surgery of the lung, or in patients receiving **positive-pressure ventilation**. The current patient had both of these predisposing conditions.

Several surgical series have reported that BPFs occur in roughly 1.5–3% of surgical resections of the lung, with the incidence of this complication rising with the amount of lung tissue resected. Thus, more BPFs occur after pneumonectomy than after lobectomy, and more develop after lobectomy than segmental resection. The chances that a patient undergoing resectional surgery will develop a BPF rises in the presence of conditions associated with poor wound healing, such as diabetes mellitus; malnutrition; radiation therapy, ongoing inflammation or infection, or devascularization at a stump site; or the presence of unresected tumor at the surgical margin. A recent review of 530 consecutive pneumonectomies reported an incidence of BPF of only 1.3%, all of which occurred in the first 15 postoperative days; 92% of surgeries were done to resect lung cancers, and all of the BPFs occurred in these patients.

BPF associated with mechanical ventilation is also a relatively uncommon event, with an incidence of probably no more than 2%. Nearly all patients who develop a BPF while on mechanical ventilation have severe underlying lung disease, such as adult respiratory distress syndrome (ARDS), and the mortality in such cases is extremely high.

Consequences of BPF may include a worsening of gas exchange and loss of effective tidal volume due to atelectasis and ventilation/perfusion mismatching, and infection of the pleural space from infected secretions passing through the fistula. **Closure** of the BPF is essential to avoid these problems. The first step in management is to place a chest tube, if one is not already in place, and apply suction. However, if bubbles are seen passing through the water seal for more than 24 hours after placement of the tube, a persistent air leak and BPF are present, and further intervention is required. In patients who develop a BPF without prior surgery, removing the positive-pressure ventilation should be beneficial, but this is often not possible because of underlying lung disease. Management also should involve as little positive endexpiratory pressure as possible. Various other ventilatory strategies have been advocated, including single-lung ventilation and high-frequency jet ventilation (HFJV). Experience with HFJV seems to indicate that this technique is most useful in traumatic or surgically-related BPFs; in BPFs occurring in the setting of ARDS, HFJV has been associated with a worsening of the air leak.

Direct attempts to close the fistula include the use of tissue glue, video-assisted thoracotomy with repair of the exposed bronchial stump, and open thoracotomy with surgical repair. These strategies are likely to be more successful in patients with BPFs complicating surgery. The present patient ultimately required surgical closure of his bronchial stump after which he was removed from mechanical ventilation.

Clinical Pearls

1. Low returned tidal volume and worsening gas exchange should suggest the possibility of a bronchopleural fistula (BPF) in a mechanically-ventilated patient.

2. After placement of a chest tube, treatment of BPF associated with underlying adult respiratory distress syndrome should focus on the underlying cause of the respiratory illness.

3. A variety of ventilatory strategies, including single-lung ventilation and high-frequency jet ventilation, may be used in traumatic BPF. Postsurgical BPF may require further surgical intervention to remove infected, devitalized, or residual malignant tissue.

REFERENCES

1. Al-Kattan K, Cattalani L, Goldstraw P. Bronchopleural fistula after pneumonectomy with a hand suture technique. Ann Thorac Surg 1994;58:1433–1436.
2. Sabanathan S, Richardson J. Management of postpneumonectomy bronchopleural fistulae. J Cardiovasc Surg 1994;35:449–457.
3. Asamura H, Naruke T, Tsuchiya R, et al. Bronchopleural fistulas associated with lung cancer operations: Univariate and multivariate analysis of risk factors, management, and outcome. J Thorac Cardiovasc Surg 1992;104:1456–1464.
4. Baumann NH, Sahn SA. Medical management and therapy of bronchopleural fistulas in the mechanically ventilated patient. Chest 1990;97:721–728.

PATIENT 22

A 58-year-old man with difficulty breathing and a history of multiple intubations

A 58-year-old man with a history of hypertension and ischemic cardiomyopathy was evaluated for respiratory distress that developed shortly after extubation. The patient had a history of repeated intubations for pulmonary edema and had been extubated yet again 12 hours prior to his current episode of dyspnea. Medications included furosemide, digoxin, nifedipine, atenolol, cimetidine, and Mylanta.

Physical Examination: Temperature 98°; pulse 106; respirations 30; blood pressure 160/100. Chest: equal air entry with stridor heard over the trachea. Cardiac: regular rate and rhythm, without murmurs, gallops, rubs, or jugular venous distension. Abdomen: soft, without masses or organomegaly. Neurologic: alert and oriented. Extremities: ++ pedal edema.

Laboratory Findings: WBC 12,100/μl, Hct 34.9%. Na$^+$ 139 mEq/L, K$^+$ 5.9 mEq/L, Cl$^-$ 98 mEq/L, HCO$_3^-$ 29 mEq/L, TCO$_2$ 30 mEq/L. ABG (non-rebreathing mask): pH 7.36, pCO$_2$ 56 mmHg, pO$_2$ 328 mmHg, SaO$_2$ 99%. Chest radiograph (see below left): cardiomegaly.

Hospital Course: Despite resolution of the pulmonary edema and a clear chest radiograph, the patient complained of difficulty breathing over the subsequent 2 weeks. Blood, urine, and sputum cultures were negative. Attempts to alleviate the dyspnea through the use of bronchodilators proved unsuccessful. Thoracic CT scan (see below right): narrowing of the trachea just distal to the position of the tracheostomy, approximately 4–5 cm above the carina. PFT: FVC 2.41 L (71% predicted), FEV$_1$ 1.98 L (74% predicted), FEV$_3$ 2.35 L (73% predicted), PEFR 2.63 L/SEC (39% predicted), FEF$_{25-75}$ 1.71 L/SEC (28% predicted), IC 2.18 L (64% predicted), FRC 1.89 L (75% predicted), TLC 4.04 L (68% predicted). The dyspnea worsened, accessory muscle utilization was noted, vesicular wheezing developed, and stridor became apparent over the trachea. Intubation was attempted via direct laryngoscopy, but the endotracheal tube could not be advanced past the level of the vocal cords. As a result the patient underwent a tracheotomy in the OR.

Questions: What is the most likely cause of the patient's difficulty breathing? What are the respiratory considerations in the management of this patient?

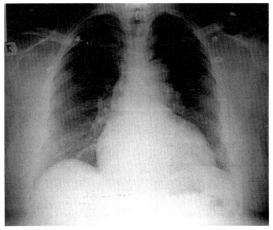
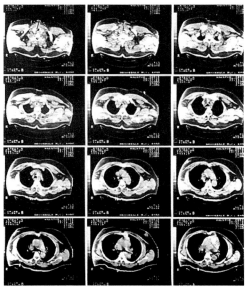

Diagnosis: Tracheomalacia with tracheal stenosis.

Discussion: Even when used properly, all endotracheal and tracheostomy tubes are potentially injurious to the patient. Most serious complications associated with these tubes are related to direct tracheal injury from excessive cuff pressures with or without systemic hypoperfusion. Typically, tracheal irritation begins at the site of the cuff and progresses to ulceration and exposure of tracheal rings, followed by fragmentation of softened cartilage and tracheal instability at the cuff site. If unchecked, the tracheostomy tube can erode anteriorly into the innominate artery and cause hemorrhage, or posteriorly through the esophagus and cause a tracheoesophageal fistula.

Tracheomalacia and tracheal stenosis are two complications that can occur separately or together. Tracheomalacia is a **softening of the cartilaginous rings** that results in the collapse of the trachea during inspiration. Processes similar to those that cause mucosal ulceration can lead to debridement of the epithelium and exposure and necrosis of the cartilaginous rings. The extent of tracheomalacia depends on the degree of cartilaginous damage. Fortunately, tracheomalacia rarely is seen in patients with translaryngeal intubation alone, not followed by tracheostomy.

Tracheal stenosis is a **narrowing of the tracheal lumen** that can occur as the tracheal rings begin the healing process. Fibrous scarring causes the airway to narrow. In patients with endotracheal tubes, this type of damage usually occurs as a result of circumferential ulceration caused by the tube cuff, but may not be evident until long after extubation and discharge. In patients with tracheostomy tubes, stenosis may occur at the cuff site or the tip of the tube, but most often at the stoma. This stenosis may be caused by too large a stoma, infection of the stoma, movement of the tube, or frequent tube changes.

Signs of possible tracheal damage prior to extubation include difficulty in sealing the trachea with the cuff and evidence of tracheal dilatation on radiographic film. Signs and symptoms following extubation include difficulty with expectoration, dyspnea at rest, and stridor. **Pulmonary function studies** may be helpful in quantifying the severity of tracheal involvement. Tracheomalacia appears as a variable, extrathoracic obstruction with flattening of the inspiratory portion of the flow volume. Tracheal stenosis appears as a fixed obstructive pattern with flattening of both the inspiratory and expiratory limbs of the flow-volume loop.

Prevention is dependent on adherence to accepted principles of airway management. Skill in intubation techniques, selection of properly designed tubes and adapters, and monitoring of tracheal tube cuff pressures are critical aspects of care. Perfusion pressure of the tracheal mucosa ranges from 18–30 mmHg. The use of minimal leak technique or minimal occluding volume as a means of cuff inflation ensures that pressures are kept well below those levels. Most importantly, prolonged intubation should be avoided whenever possible.

Treatment depends on the severity of the damage, especially the length and circumference of the involved area. For stenotic lesions causing < 25% narrowing of the airway lumen, no treatment may be necessary, and a period of observation is justified. Laser therapy can be useful if the lesion is small. Resection and end-to-end anastomosis may be indicated when the damage involves less than three tracheal rings. More extensive damage generally requires staged surgical repair.

Because of the stridor and respiratory difficulty the present patient was experiencing, a tracheostomy was performed, after which the patient underwent a successful laser resection of the stenosis.

Clinical Pearls

1. Symptoms of tracheal stenosis may not be noticeable, except by pulmonary function tests, until the stricture reduces tracheal diameter by as much as 50%.
2. Stridor typically does not occur until the tracheal lumen is < 5 mm in diameter.
3. Use, monitoring, and care of appropriately sized, high residual volume, low-pressure tracheal tubes are essential in the prevention of tracheal abnormalities such as malacia and stenosis.

REFERENCES

1. Yang KL. Tracheal stenosis after a brief intubation. Anesth Analg 1995;80:625–627.
2. Grillo HC, Donahue DM, Mathisen DJ, et al. Postintubation tracheal stenosis: Treatment and results. J Thorac Cardiovasc Surg 1995;109:486–492.
3. Whitehead E, Salam MA. Use of the carbon dioxide laser with the Montgomery T-tube in the management of extensive subglottic stenosis. J Laryngol Otol 1992;106:829–831.

PATIENT 23

A 28-week gestational age, 700-gram infant girl with paradoxical respirations and severe respiratory distress

A 28-week gestational age, 700-gram infant girl was born to a mother who had received no prenatal care. The mother's course of labor was preceded by early rupture of amniotic membranes and complicated by vaginal hemorrhage; the infant was born by vaginal delivery.

Physical Examination: Temperature 93.2°; pulse 173; respirations 29; blood pressure 38/22. Apgar score 6,7. Chest: suprasternal, substernal, and intercostal retractions; audible expiratory grunting. Extremities: central cyanosis.

Laboratory Findings: WBC 9,300/μl, Hct 47%. Na$^+$ 133 mEq/L, K$^+$ 4.6 mEq/L, Cl$^-$ 99 mEq/L. Glucose 82 mg/dl, BUN 8 mg/dl, Cr 0.3 mg/dl. Chest radiograph (see below): hazy bilateral lung densities most pronounced near the hila.

Hospital Course: The infant was intubated at eight minutes using a 2.5 mm uncuffed endotracheal tube. She was transferred to the neonatal intensive care unit and mechanical ventilation was initiated using a BEAR BP-200 ventilator with the following settings: PIP 18 cm H$_2$O, f = 40 IPPB/IMV, FiO$_2$ 1.0, PEEP of 5 cm H$_2$O, and a set flow rate of 10 L/min. Resultant ABG: pH 7.31, pCO$_2$ 48 mmHg, pO$_2$ 113 mmHg, HCO$_3^-$ 24 mEq/L, SaO$_2$ 97%.

Questions: What is the most likely diagnosis in this patient? What are the respiratory care considerations in the management of this disease?

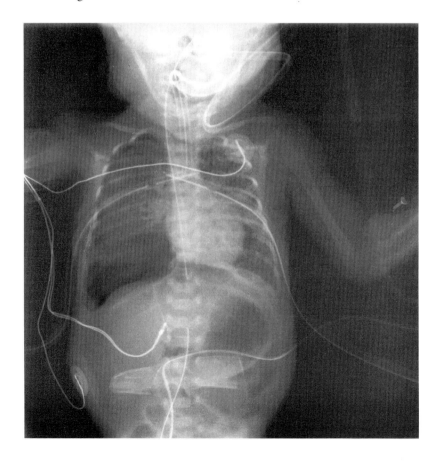

Diagnosis: Hyaline membrane disease (infant respiratory distress syndrome).

Discussion: Hyaline membrane disease (HMD) is one of the most common causes of severe respiratory distress in newborns. Its occurrence relates directly to the gestational age of the infant, as well as to the birthweight. Roughly half of all infants born at < 28 weeks of gestation develop this complication, and none of those reaching full-term are affected. Similarly, about one-seventh of infants weighing < 2500 grams are affected.

The etiology of HMD is related to **abnormalities of surfactant function** in the immature lung. Primarily, there seems to be an abnormality of the lipid component of surfactant, most importantly in the function of desaturated phosphatidylcholine (DSPC), which can be predicted by measuring the ratio of lecithin (L) to sphingomyelin (S) in amniotic fluid before birth. The concentration of lecithin (the major functional lipid portion of surfactant), of which DSPC is a component, should increase continually throughout gestation, as compared with the concentration of sphingomyelin, which remains stable in amniotic fluid during pregnancy. By the 32nd week of gestation in a normal pregnancy, the L/S ratio is about 1.0, and it rises to 2.0 usually by the 35th week of gestation. At a L/S ratio of 2.0 or greater, the risk of developing HMD is about 1 in 200, whereas the incidence rises to essentially 100% for ratios below 1.0. Even in patients with ratios above 2.0, HMD may occur if the concentration of phosphatidylglycerine is low.

The sequelae of inadequate surfactant function at birth are fairly predictable. Atelectasis, ventilation/perfusion mismatching, shunting, reduced lung compliance, and a low functional reserve capacity (FRC) all contribute to the respiratory distress and gas exchange abnormalities which characterize the disorder. Mechanical ventilation is required for a significant number of infants born with HMD, and the long-term consequences of artificial respiration include bronchopulmonary dysplasia, which can be crippling.

Treatment of HMD falls into two categories: prenatal and postpartum. Before birth, if the risk of HMD is high as predicted by a low L/S ratio, administration of **corticosteroids** can accelerate surfactant maturation and reduce risk, although treatment generally must begin 24–48 hours before birth. After birth, **oxygen therapy** and **mechanical ventilation** are applied as needed, though the risks and adverse effects associated with these therapies can be substantial.

In recent years, **surfactant replacement therapy** has come to play a major role in the treatment of HMD. Initial controlled clinical studies of exogenous surfactant administration demonstrated significant improvements in gas exchange, FRC, and lung compliance, and pathologic studies showed significantly less advanced hyaline membrane formation, pulmonary interstitial emphysema, and epithelial necrosis. Surfactant administration has come into wide use for low birth-weight babies. Several large studies have now demonstrated 30–40% reductions in mortality among very low birth-weight babies (those weighing 500–1500 grams) treated with exogenous surfactant immediately after birth.

The most recent development in the treatment of infant respiratory distress syndrome is the use of **partial-liquid ventilation**. In this approach, a perfluorocarbon liquid with a large carrying capacity for oxygen is administered intratracheally to infants with HMD. A recent study of this approach in infants who were failing all conventional therapy, including surfactant administration, demonstrated rapid improvements in oxygenation and dynamic compliance, with survival in 8 of 10 infants studied. Wider use of this technique awaits larger trials.

The infant in this case was supported successfully for nine weeks following endobronchial instillation of an exogenous, modified, natural surfactant preparation. Improvements were noted in compliance, oxygenation, and chest radiography. She was weaned to extubation and discharged two weeks following discontinuation of ventilatory support.

Clinical Pearls

1. Prediction of the development of hyaline membrane disease (HMD) can be aided by measuring the lecithin/sphingomyelin ratio in amniotic fluid, with HMD likely at ratios below 1.0 and excluded for ratios above 2.0.

2. The incidence and severity of infant respiratory distress syndrome (HMD) can be reduced if the mother of a fetus known to be at risk is given corticosteroids 48 hours prior to delivery.

3. Administration of exogenous surfactant immediately after birth to infants at risk for HMD results in substantially decreased morbidity and mortality.

REFERENCES

1. Leach CL, Greenspan JS, Rubinstein SD, et al. Partial liquid ventilation with perfluorocarbon in premature infants with severe respiratory distress syndrome. N Engl J Med 1996;335:761–776.
2. Schwartz RM, Luby AM, Scanlon JW, Kellogg RJ. Effect of surfactant on morbidity, mortality, and resource utilization in newborn infants weighing 500 to 1500 g. N Engl J Med 1994;330:1476–1480.
3. Pfenninger J, Aebi C, Bachmann D, Wagner BP. Lung mechanics and gas exchange in ventilated preterm infants during treatment of hyaline membrane disease with multiple doses of artificial surfactant. Pediatr Pulmonol 1992;14:10–15.
4. Bartholomew KM, Brownlee KG, Snowden S, Dear PR. To PEEP or not to PEEP? Arch Dis Child 1994;70:F209–212.

PATIENT 24

A 45-year-old man with possible drug overdose and respiratory depression

A 45-year-old man was found unresponsive at home by paramedics after an apparent suicide attempt. Past medical history included repeated suicide attempts as well as asthma, hypertension, and depression. Medications included captopril, nifedipine, amitriptyline, diazepam, and metaproterenol.

Physical Examination: Temperature 99°; pulse 105; respirations 8; blood pressure 114/70. Chest: clear to auscultation. Neurologic: unresponsive with a Glasgow Coma Scale score of 6; pupils bilaterally constricted.

Laboratory Findings: WBC 14,220/μl with 84.8% neutrophils, 5.8% lymphocytes. K^+ 3.4 mEq/L, glucose 116 mg/dl, ALT 20 IU/L, PT 12.8 sec, PTT 21.2 sec, control 11.0 sec. ABG (room air): pH 7.3, pCO_2 48 mmHg, pO_2 75 mmHg, HCO_3^- 24 mEq/L. Chest radiograph (see below).

Questions: What is the most probable cause of the patient's respiratory depression? What are the initial respiratory considerations in the care of this patient?

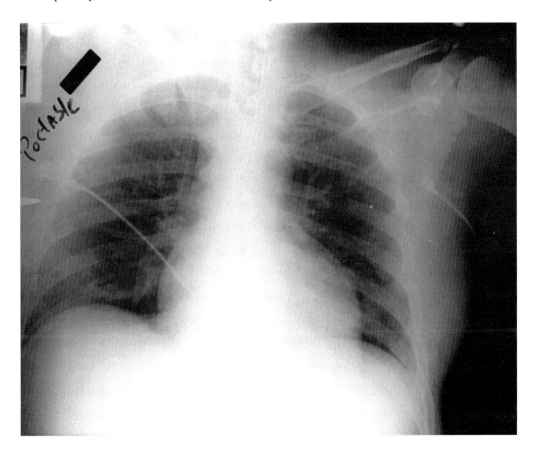

Diagnosis: Ventilatory failure due to polypharmacy intoxication.

Discussion: Sedative-hypnotics and antidepressants are among the most widely used drugs in the United States today, and physicians and other health care professionals working in respiratory care units must be familiar with their use and abuse. Of the sedative-hypnotic agents, **benzodiazepines** remain the most ubiquitous, and although they are generally safe and unlikely to cause a fatal drug overdose on their own, they can be associated with significant respiratory depression. These drugs act on receptors in the central nervous system, increasing their affinity for gamma-aminobutyric acid (GABA), an inhibitory neurotransmitter. With increased GABA binding, decreased CNS function and depressed consciousness ensue.

Usually, significant cardiovascular and respiratory effects do not accompany the therapeutic agents for depression and/or anxiolysis. However, these effects are commonly seen when large doses of benzodiazepines are given. Blood pressure and cardiac output can drop as much as 15% after a dose of midazolam large enough to induce general anesthesia (or as might be delivered in an overdose). In addition, benzodiazepines can cause respiratory depression by impairing ventilatory responses to hypercarbia and hypoxemia, both of which can become quite severe at high blood levels of benzodiazepines.

In general, ventilatory depression following ingestion of **antidepressants** is a much less significant clinical problem than with benzodiazepines. Effects of tricyclic antidepressants are generally related to one of four mechanisms: anticholinergic action, sodium channel blockade, prevention of reuptake of neurotransmitters such as norepinephrine, serotonin, and dopamine, and blockade of α-adrenergic receptors. Of these, cardiac electrophysiologic effects related to sodium channel blockade are potentially the most lethal and include QT prolongation and QRS complex widening, which can lead to lethal arrhythmias. Seizure activity, often treated with benzodiazepines, can also occur.

The newer antidepressants, such as fluoxetine, are inhibitors of serotonin reuptake and appear to have far fewer serious side effects than the tricyclic agents. Significant respiratory depression probably does not occur with fluoxetine.

General principles of respiratory care for patients with sedative and/or antidepressant overdose are identical to those for managing overdoses and ingestions of other agents. These principles are discussed elsewhere in this volume (see Patient 9). However, note should be made of flumazenil, a short-acting, benzodiazepine antagonist capable of reversing the depression of consciousness associated with benzodiazepine administration. Although flumazenil has come into wide use over the past few years, for a variety of reasons it is *not* recommended for routine therapy in patients with benzodiazepine overdose. Flumazenil has a much shorter half-life and duration of action than most of the benzodiazepines prescribed in clinical practice, so that even if respiratory status transiently improved after its administration, the patient might quickly slip back into respiratory failure. Additionally, flumazenil may induce a syndrome of benzodiazepine withdrawal accompanied by nausea and vomiting and can even cause seizures in patients receiving cyclic antidepressants such as fluoxetine. Thus, a diagnostic dose of flumazenil might be helpful in determining if benzodiazepines are contributing to a patient's depressed consciousness, but routine administration in coma is to be discouraged.

The current patient required intubation and mechanical ventilation for respiratory depression. He was treated with supportive care and was extubated 48 hours after admission. He was then transferred to the psychiatric service for further care.

Clinical Pearls

1. Of the commonly used sedative hypnotics and antidepressants, benzodiazepines are most often associated with respiratory depression when taken in large doses or in suicide attempts.

2. Therapy for overdose of benzodiazepines is largely supportive and follows the principles of care for poisonings in general. In general, mortality from benzodiazepine overdose should be quite low.

3. The specific benzodiazepine antagonist flumazenil has a short duration of action and can provoke the syndrome of benzodiazepine withdrawal. It should not be used therapeutically to routinely treat benzodiazepine overdose.

REFERENCES
1. Foulke GE. Identifying toxicity risk early after antidepressant overdose. Am J Emerg Med 1995;13:123–126.
2. Hoffman RS, Goldfrank LR. The poisoned patient with altered consciousness. Controversies in the use of a "coma cocktail." JAMA 1995;274:562–569.
3. Shalansky SJ, Naumann TL, Englander FA. Effect of flumazenil on benzodiazepine-induced respiratory depression. Clin Pharmacy 1993;12:483–487.

PATIENT 25

**A 68-year-old man with chronic obstructive pulmonary disease
and progressive dyspnea**

A 68-year-old man with a past medical history of COPD complicated by cor pulmonale presented to his physician's office with progressive shortness of breath. He had been able to walk up to 15 feet without difficulty until 3 weeks previously when his dyspnea worsened to the point that he was short of breath at rest. Current medications included theophylline, furosemide, continuous oxygen via nasal cannula at 2 L/min, and albuterol and triamcinolone via metered-dose inhalers.

Physical Examination: Temperature 99.7°; pulse 92; respirations 26 with accessory muscle use noted; blood pressure 150/85. Chest: diminished breath sounds at the bases with basilar rales. Cardiac: regular rate and rhythm, JVD and right-sided S_3 noted. Abdomen: soft, without masses or organomegaly. Neurologic: alert and oriented, nonfocal exam. Extremities: +++ pedal edema.

Laboratory Findings: WBC 12,200/μl, Hct 57.6%. K^+ 3.5 mEq/L, Cl^- 90 mEq/L, HCO_3^- 31 mEq/L. ABG (O_2 2 L/min): pH 7.34, pCO_2 58 mmHg, pO_2 46 mmHg, SaO_2 77%. Chest radiograph (see below): marked hyperinflation of the lung fields, with blunting of the right costophrenic angle and flattened diaphragms.

Questions: What is the most likely diagnosis in this patient? What is the role of noninvasive ventilation in this patient?

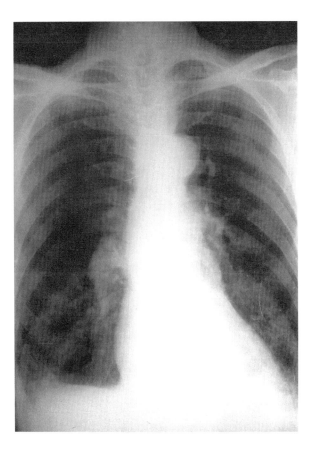

Diagnosis: Acute exacerbation of chronic obstructive lung disease with cor pulmonale.

Discussion: When a patient with COPD presents with a worsening respiratory status, it can be difficult to determine the exact cause of the decompensation. In general, the major diagnostic considerations include a respiratory infection (which may be something as seemingly trivial as a viral bronchitis); a cardiac problem such as congestive heart failure, the radiographic pattern of which may be somewhat atypical in a patient with severe underlying emphysema; or pulmonary embolism, particularly if the patient has been restricted to bed owing to the underlying pulmonary insufficiency. In addition, noncompliance with medical therapy, particularly in patients with severe COPD requiring home oxygen therapy, may contribute to a worsening status.

In patients with acute exacerbations of COPD, whatever the specific cause of the deterioration, the ultimately physiologic consequence is similar: additional stress is placed on an already severely stressed respiratory pump. The **oxygen cost of breathing** (the fraction of oxygen consumption or total cardiac output needed to fuel the respiratory muscles), is higher than normal in patients with COPD, due in part to altered chest wall anatomy, abnormal length-tension relationships of the respiratory muscles, loss of elastic recoil (characteristic of emphysema), and increased airways resistance caused by bronchial wall thickening and secretions (typical in chronic bronchitis). This already high oxygen cost becomes substantially higher during exacerbations.

In healthy individuals, the oxygen cost of breathing accounts for < 5% of total oxygen consumption; in COPD patients it can rise to 15–20% of total O_2 consumption. Moreover, several studies have indicated that in COPD patients receiving mechanical ventilation, the O_2 cost of breathing may rise as high as 50% of total O_2 consumption. The excessive respiratory muscle workload is a substantial barrier to recovery—the respiratory muscles must be rested to allow enough fuel for the body to address the problem underlying the exacerbation.

In recent years, the use of noninvasive, positive-pressure ventilation as a means of providing ventilatory support to COPD patients with acute respiratory failure while at the same time **resting respiratory muscles** has been intensively investigated. In one study of inpatients treated for COPD, the spontaneous oxygen cost of breathing was found to be 15% of total O_2 consumption, nearly four times higher than that found for normal volunteers. After application of continuous positive airway pressure (CPAP), the oxygen cost of breathing fell to 9% of total O_2 consumption. In another study of nasal CPAP to treat COPD it was found that nocturnal applications of noninvasive ventilation apparently could allow enough rest during inspiratory muscle activity to improve inspiratory muscle strength and endurance during wakefulness. In settings of acute respiratory failure complicating COPD, the application of CPAP was found to improve gas exchange and reduce diaphragmatic effort to a degree similar to that achieved with pressure-support ventilation and PEEP.

Only a few controlled trials of noninvasive ventilation for acute exacerbations of COPD have been done. Still, it seems reasonable to attempt this mode of ventilatory support in patients with hypercarbic respiratory failure who are awake and alert enough to cooperate and who are not in need of frequent suctioning to control secretions. In such patients, noninvasive strategies for ventilation may obviate the need for intubation and mechanical ventilation and reduce morbidity related to those procedures.

The current patient was treated with oxygen, bronchodilators, diuretics, and antibiotics. He improved without requiring ventilatory assistance and was discharged home on continuous oxygen therapy.

Clinical Pearls

1. Though acute decompensation in COPD is often due to a seemingly mild respiratory illness or infection, congestive heart failure and pulmonary embolism must also be considered in the differential diagnosis.

2. During exacerbations of COPD, the respiratory muscles may require 15–40% of the body's total oxygen consumption.

3. Noninvasive strategies of ventilation, such as the application of CPAP via mask, may reduce the need for mechanical ventilation in selected patients.

REFERENCES

1. Weyland W, Schuhmann M, Rathgeber J, et al. Oxygen cost of breathing for assisted spontaneous breathing modes: Investigation into three states of pulmonary function. Intens Care Med 1995;21:211–217.
2. Mezzanotte WS, Tangel DJ, Fox AM, et al. Nocturnal nasal continuous positive airway pressure in patients with chronic obstructive pulmonary disease. Influence on waking respiratory muscle function. Chest 1994;106:1100–1108.
3. Appendini L, Patessioj A, Zanaboni S, et al. Physiologic effects of positive end-expiratory pressure and mask pressure support during exacerbations of chronic obstructive pulmonary disease. Am J Respir Crit Care Med 1994:149:1069–1076.
4. MacNee W. Pathophysiology of cor pulmonale in chronic obstructive pulmonary disease. Am J Respir Crit Care Med 1994;150:833–852.
5. Emerman CL, Cydulka RK. Evaluation of high-yield criteria for chest radiography in acute exacerbation of chronic obstructive pulmonary disease. Ann Emerg Med 1993;22:680–684.
6. Jeffrey AA, Warren PM, Flenley DC. Acute hypercapnic respiratory failure in patients with chronic obstructive lung disease: Risk factors and use of guidelines for management. Thorax 1992;47:34–40.

PATIENT 26

A 73-year-old woman with cough, hoarseness, and dizziness

A 73-year-old woman was brought to the emergency department with cough, hoarseness, and dizziness after being exposed to smoke from a fire. Past medical history included hypertension, arthritis, and a cerebrovascular accident.

Physical Examination: Temperature 98.2°; pulse 80; respirations 22; blood pressure 210/90. HEENT: no singed nasal hairs or eyebrows noted. Chest: clear to auscultation, without wheezes. Cardiac: regular rhythm, without murmurs. Abdomen: soft, nontender, without organomegaly. Extremities: no cyanosis or edema. Neurologic: nonfocal exam, though patient complaining of dizziness.

Laboratory Findings: Na^+ 145 mEq/L, K^+ 3.3 mEq/L, ionized calcium 4.8 mg/dL. ABG (nonrebreathing mask): pH 7.44, pCO_2 37 mmHg, pO_2 86 mmHg, HCO_3^- 25 mEq/L, SaO_2 97%. Carboxyhemoglobin: 25%. Chest radiograph: see below.

Hospital Course: While receiving oxygen therapy, the patient began to manifest signs and symptoms of neurological inappropriateness, including confusion and amnesia. Lung sounds demonstrated diffuse wheezes which responded to nebulized albuterol. Repeat ABG: pH 7.42, pCO_2 41 mmHg, pO_2 66 mmHg, HCO_3^- 27 mEq/L, SaO_2 94%.

Questions: What is the most likely diagnosis in this patient? What are the respiratory considerations in the management of this patient?

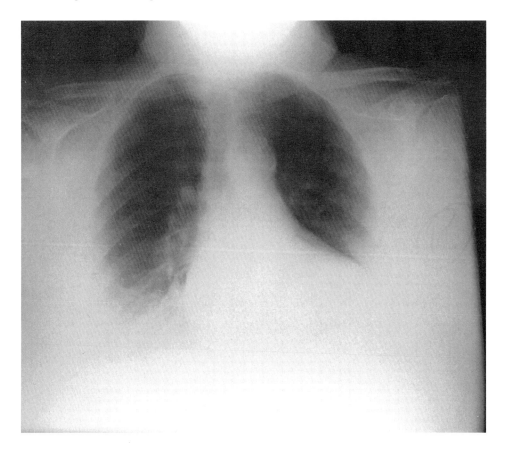

Diagnosis: Smoke inhalation with carbon monoxide poisoning.

Discussion: Persons exposed to fire and smoke are susceptible to injury in a variety of ways, and the respiratory care implications are related to each of the potential mechanisms of injury. The most direct mechanism of injury is a burn to the respiratory tract by the inhalation of **hot smoke or particulates**. In most instances, the nasopharynx and oropharynx are efficient heat exchangers so that severe burns to the lower respiratory tract are not commonly seen. The exception is steam inhalation, as steam has a much higher heat capacitance than most other inhaled substances.

The consequences of thermal injury are edema and necrosis of the respiratory epithelium, which can result in severe tracheal edema and obstruction. Clues to the presence of a thermal burn to the respiratory tract include singed nasal hairs or eyebrows. For severe airway burns, intubation may be required so that fatal airway obstruction does not occur. Prophylactic use of steroids in this setting has not been demonstrated to be beneficial and may be associated with a higher risk of superinfection.

The second type of injury that can be sustained in a fire results from the toxic effects of the **products of combustion**. The list of toxic substances produced during combustion in a typical household fire is long and includes agents such as acrolein, ammonia, chlorine, phosgene, hydrogen chloride, and trimellitic anhydride—all of which can produce severe chemical burns throughout the respiratory tree, bronchospasm, and adult respiratory distress syndrome (ARDS). When taking a history or surveying a fire scene, all substances involved in the fire should be noted for clues to toxic combustion products. The delayed onset of ARDS may complicate these exposures.

The third type of injury associated with smoke inhalation is **carbon monoxide (CO) poisoning**.

CO can cause asphyxiation because of its great affinity for oxygen, to which it binds 250 times more avidly than hemoglobin. CO displaces oxygen from hemoglobin, shifts the oxyhemoglobin dissociation curve to the left, and depresses cellular respiration by the inhibition of cytochrome a_3 oxidase. The net effect can be profound tissue hypoxia, anaerobic metabolism, and lactic acidosis. The toxic effects of CO poisoning include those seen as a result of hypoxia in any tissue, such as myocardial ischemia and a variety of CNS effects.

Symptoms and morbidity from CO poisoning directly correlate with the CO level. (Interestingly, smokers often have carboxyhemoglobin (COHb) levels around 10%. COHb levels at 20–40% are associated with dizziness, headache, weakness, nausea and vomiting, and diminished visual acuity. Levels at 40–60% generally produce tachypnea, tachycardia, ataxia, syncope, and the precipitation of seizures. Levels above 60% often result in coma and death.

Treatment of CO poisoning includes supportive care and the routine initial administration of 100% oxygen. Supplemental oxygen therapy ensures tissue oxygen delivery while decreasing CO half-life. The half-lives of CO in room air, 100% oxygen, and 100% oxygen at three atmospheres are 4–5 hours, 90 minutes, and 23 minutes, respectively. Hyperbaric oxygen support is strongly recommended for patients who present with neurologic deficits, electrocardiographic changes suggestive of ischemia, severe metabolic acidosis, pulmonary edema, or shock. Transfer to a hyperbaric facility should occur only after the patient is stabilized.

The present patient was stabilized, treated with oxygen therapy, and referred to a hyperbaric facility via air transfer because of her COHb level, presenting symptoms, and past medical history.

Clinical Pearls

1. Management of the patient with smoke inhalation requires assessment of the airway for thermal injury as well as toxic injury from the products of combustion and examination for carbon monoxide (CO) poisoning.

2. Because arterial PO_2 may be normal with CO poisoning, definitive diagnosis requires a high index of suspicion and direct measurement of carboxyhemoglobin (COHb) levels.

3. All patients with elevated COHb levels should receive 100% oxygen. Hyperbaric therapy is indicated for any elevation of COHb with symptoms of end-organ damage, and it should be considered for any patient with a level above 25%.

REFERENCES

1. Shimada H, Morita T, Kunimoto F, Saito S. Immediate application of hyperbaric oxygen therapy using a newly devised transportable chamber. Am J Emerg Med 1996;14:412–415.
2. Shusterman D, Alexeeff G, Hargis C, et al. Predictors of carbon monoxide and hydrogen cyanide exposure in smoke inhalation patients. J Toxicol Clin Toxicol 1996;34:61–71.
3. Wittram C, Kenny JB. The admission chest radiograph after acute inhalation injury and burns. Brit J Radiol 1994;67:751–754.
4. Hollingsed TC, Saffle JR, Barton RG, et al. Etiology and consequences of respiratory failure in thermally injured patients. Am J Surg 1993;166:592–596.

PATIENT 27

A 52-year-old man with ventilator dependence for 8 months

A 52-year-old man with amyotrophic lateral sclerosis was admitted to the chronic ventilator unit of a chronic-care nursing facility. He had been receiving mechanical ventilatory support for the past 8 months for progressive muscle weakness.

Physical Examination: Temperature 98.6°; pulse 78; respirations 16, assisted; blood pressure 104/70. Chest: without rhonchi or wheezes. Cardiac: regular rate and rhythm, without murmurs. Abdomen: soft, nontender, with percutaneous gastrostomy tube in place. Extremities: no cyanosis, clubbing, or edema. Neurologic: alert and oriented; marked motor weakness, 1–2/5 strength and flaccidity throughout.

Laboratory Findings: Na^+ 138 mEq/L, K^+ 4.0 mEq/L, Cl^- 99 mEq/L, HCO_3^- 27 mEq/L. Glucose 93 mg/dl, BUN 21 mg/dl, Cr 0.4 mg/dl. Admission ABG (FiO_2 0.3): pH 7.53, pCO_2 32 mmHg, pO_2 99 mmHg, SaO_2 98%. Chest radiograph: see below.

Questions: What are the physiologic correlates of respiratory failure in amyotrophic lateral sclerosis? What alternative strategies for ventilatory assistance are available for this patient?

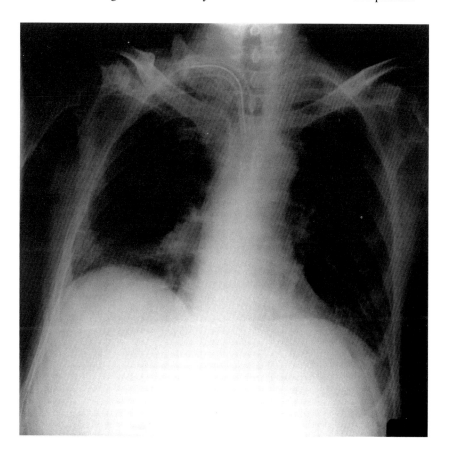

Diagnosis: Chronic respiratory failure due to amyotrophic lateral sclerosis (ALS).

Discussion: Though less common than other causes of chronic ventilatory failure, neuromuscular diseases pose a challenging set of problems in respiratory care. As a group, they are a heterogeneous collection that affects respiratory function primarily via central ventilatory drive (central sleep apnea and other disorders of automatic respiration) or respiratory muscle strength. ALS is one of several diseases associated mainly with **muscle weakness** that cause atrophy of all skeletal muscle through chronic denervation resulting from chronic degeneration of upper and lower motor neurons. Other diseases in this class include Guillain-Barré syndrome (ascending inflammatory polyneuropathy) and myasthenia gravis, in which antibodies to acetylcholine receptors cause muscle weakness because of ineffective neurotransmission.

ALS is the most common form of **progressive motor neuron disease**. It is a prototypical example of a neuronal system disease and can be considered the most devastating of the neurodegenerative disorders. As there is no specific therapy, most patients will eventually develop respiratory failure, owing primarily to diaphragmatic weakness. The respiratory failure is manifested by a steadily falling vital capacity (VC) throughout the course of the disease, until adequate ventilation can no longer be sustained. Accompanying the fall in VC is a corresponding decline in maximum voluntary ventilation (MVV). Though obstruction to airflow is not a feature of neuromuscular diseases, the residual volume (RV) in ALS is elevated because of a reduction in expired air associated with intercostal and abdominal muscle weakness. Functional residual capacity (FRC) is also diminished and, importantly, the mean inspiratory and expiratory pressures (MIP, MEP) are decreased. Chest wall and total lung compliance typically are normal to increased.

The consequences of these abnormalities lead directly to ventilatory failure in ALS patients. Progressive muscle weakness eventually leads to hypercapnic respiratory failure, usually when the VC falls below 1 L. Often accompanying this fall in VC is an ineffective cough mechanism, related to the low MIP and MEP, that can lead to a problem clearing secretions and the development of pneumonia.

Ventilatory strategies for ALS patients with respiratory failure include both positive- and negative-pressure approaches. Negative-pressure approaches such as the Poncho-wrap, Pneumosuit, rocking bed, or firm chest cuirass can be successful since chest wall compliance is low, and the negative pressure generated does not have to be great to provide sufficient ventilation. However, these modes are of limited value if handling secretions is a problem. At early stages of respiratory insufficiency, nocturnal positive-pressure ventilation via nasal prongs may be used, but eventually patients require permanent support. If this approach is selected, it makes sense to perform a tracheostomy at the outset, as the need for ventilatory support will not diminish over time. A variety of home ventilators now available are capable of providing adequate respiratory support if accompanied by the proper respiratory care and nursing support.

The present patient receives continuous mechanical ventilatory support as a resident of a chronic-care facility.

Clinical Pearls

1. Amyotrophic lateral sclerosis (ALS) is a progressive, degenerative disorder of upper and lower motor neurons which generally results in neuromuscular respiratory failure in its later stages.

2. Pulmonary function abnormalities in ALS include reduced VC, MVV, MIP, MEP, as well as increased RV and slightly increased FRC. Significant respiratory failure generally occurs when the VC falls below 1 L.

3. A variety of ventilatory strategies are available to ALS patients with hypercarbic respiratory failure. Most patients, if they choose life support, require tracheostomy and positive-pressure ventilation to best provide adequate ventilation and handle secretions.

REFERENCES
1. Marti-Fabregas J, Dourado M, Sanchis J, et al. Respiratory function deterioration is not time-linked with upper-limb onset in amyotrophic lateral sclerosis. Acta Neurol Scand 1995;92:261–264.
2. Sherman MS, Paz HL. Review of respiratory care of the patient with amyotrophic lateral sclerosis. Respiration 1994;61:61–67.
3. Annane D, Korach JM, Templier F, et al. Diaphragmatic paralysis preceding amyotrophic lateral sclerosis. Lancet 1993; 342:990–991.
4. Schiffman PL, Belsh JM. Pulmonary function at diagnosis of amyotrophic lateral sclerosis. Rate of deterioration. Chest 1993; 103:508–513.

PATIENT 28

A 54-year-old woman with progressive shortness of breath for 2 days

A 54-year-old woman was brought to the emergency department with a chief complaint of breathlessness for 2 days. Her past medical history was notable for a recent diagnosis of idiopathic pulmonary fibrosis requiring continuous oxygen support at home. A pulmonary function study performed one month prior to admission revealed a severe restrictive lung disease, and she had been maintained on prednisone.

Physical Examination: Temperature 98.2°; pulse 138; respirations 30; blood pressure 120/74; height 60 inches; weight 52 kg. Chest: tachypnea with basilar dry rales and decreased breath sounds bilaterally. Cardiac: regular rhythm and rate. Abdomen: soft, nontender, without masses or organomegaly. Extremities: + clubbing. Neurologic: nonfocal.

Laboratory Findings: CBC, electrolytes: within normal limits. Room air blood gas: pH 7.44, pCO_2 33 mmHg, pO_2 44 mmHg, HCO_3^- 22 mEq/L, SaO_2 82%. Chest radiograph: see below.

Hospital Course: The patient was intubated because of hypoxemic respiratory failure. Mechanical ventilatory support was initiated with a Siemens Servo 900C ventilator with the following settings: volume control mode, V_t 650 ml, f = 16, FiO_2 1.0 and 5 cm H_2O PEEP. Repeat ABG: pH 7.28, pCO_2 42 mmHg, pO_2 62 mmHg, HCO_3^- 20 mEq/L, SaO_2 90%. Airway pressure with these settings was noted to be 66 cm H_2O. A pulmonary artery catheter was placed and yielded the following hemodynamic indices: pulmonary artery (PA) systolic pressure 54 mmHg, PA diastolic pressure 16 mmHg, mean PA pressure 35 mmHg, pulmonary artery occlusion pressure (wedge pressure) 18 mmHg. An order was then written to place the patient on inverse ratio ventilation (IRV).

Questions: What are the postulated physiologic mechanisms supporting the use of IRV? How should IRV be employed?

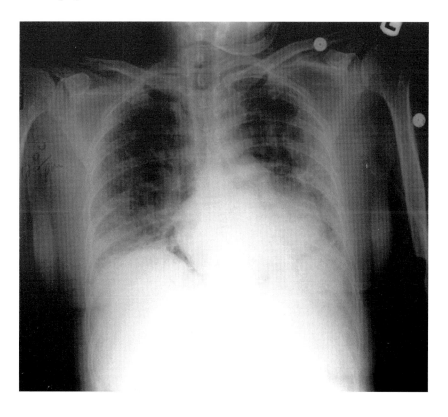

Diagnosis: Hypoxic respiratory failure and the adult respiratory distress syndrome complicating interstitial lung disease.

Discussion: Management of patients with refractory hypoxia requiring mechanical ventilation is an especially difficult clinical problem, and several ventilatory strategies have been devised in recent years to improve gas exchange in these patients. Among these, there has been considerable interest in **inverse ratio ventilation** (IRV) as a means of improving gas exchange to life-sustaining levels. Employment of this strategy requires awareness of inherent physiologic mechanisms and potential complications.

For the past several years, the standard approach to treating refractory hypoxia in patients with adult respiratory distress syndrome (ARDS) has been to apply increasing levels of positive end-expiratory pressure (PEEP) with the goal of **recruiting collapsed alveoli**. The determination of optimal or "best" PEEP has been the source of much discussion, but it is clear that deleterious effects do occur at the high levels of PEEP required in many ARDS patients. These effects include a risk of pneumothorax as well as a danger of overdistending and thereby injuring normal alveoli (so-called volutrauma). IRV has been developed as a respiratory strategy to address some of these issues and to provide adequate oxygenation in otherwise refractory cases of hypoxia.

In IRV, the normal inspiratory ratio is reversed so that the ratio of inspiration time to expiration time is typically 2:1, 3:1, or 4:1. The rationale behind this strategy is to attempt to recruit collapsed alveoli *without* overdistending normal lung units. In IRV, the mean airway pressure (MAP), which correlates, though imperfectly, with mean alveolar pressure, rises more than the peak airway pressure as long as expiratory time is sufficient and dynamic hyperinflation (auto-PEEP) is not allowed to occur. Theoretically, the corresponding rise in mean alveolar pressure causes an increase in alveolar recruitment, and gas exchange improves. In addition, IRV may allow better ventilation of the alveoli with longer time constants and may reduce dead-space ventilation by improving collateral ventilation.

IRV can be implemented with either a volume-cycled or a pressure-controlled ventilator. When using a volume-cycled ventilator, the inspiration/expiration ratio (I:E) is manipulated by adding an end-inspiratory pause to the respiratory cycle or by decreasing the inspiratory flow rate. The major advantage of using a volume-cycled ventilator for IRV is that a guaranteed tidal volume is delivered to the patient. Disadvantages of this approach include wide variations in peak airway and alveolar pressure, particularly if auto-PEEP develops or respiratory compliance changes markedly. In addition, most patients receiving volume-cycled IRV find it to be a very uncomfortable mode of mechanical ventilation, and the heavy sedation typically required is often accompanied by paralysis. In pressure-controlled IRV, the I:E ratio can be dialed in directly, and the peak airway pressure also is directly controlled and limited, reducing the risk of overinflation or barotrauma. Disadvantages of pressure-controlled IRV include no guaranteed tidal volume and perhaps less general availability than volume-cycled ventilation.

Complications of IRV can be serious and include the generation of auto-PEEP, barotrauma from high airway pressures, and drops in cardiac output (CO) as mean airway pressures rises, in a manner analogous to the effect of PEEP on CO. In addition, little data clearly show a benefit from the use of IRV in ARDS, despite the theoretical advantages. For these reasons, IRV should be considered a technique for use only when conventional ventilatory strategies have failed, and then only by experienced respiratory care personnel.

The present patient developed multi-system failure despite therapeutic and supportive interventions to treat her clinical syndrome. She expired 72 hours after admission to the ICU.

Clinical Pearls

1. Inverse ratio ventilation (IRV) may improve oxygenation by increasing mean alveolar pressure, by overcoming differences in time constants between ventilatory units, or by improving collateral ventilation.

2. IRV can be instituted with either volume-cycled ventilators, which guarantee tidal volume but increase the risk of high airway and alveolar pressure and require greater sedation, or pressure-cycled ventilators, which allow easier manipulation of the I:E ratio but no guaranteed tidal volume.

3. No data exist showing a definitive advantage of IRV in ARDS, and it should not be used routinely to replace conventional approaches to mechanical ventilation.

REFERENCES

1. Effros RM, Presberg K. Does inverse ratio ventilation predispose to pulmonary edema? Chest 1996;110:314–316.
2. Marini JJ. Inverse ratio ventilation—simply an alternative, or something more? Crit Care Med 1995;23:224–228.
3. Armstrong BW Jr, MacIntyre NR. Pressure-controlled, inverse ratio ventilation that avoids air trapping in the adult respiratory distress syndrome. Crit Care Med 1995;23:279–285.
4. Lessard MR, Guerot E, Lorino H, et al. Effects of pressure-controlled with different I:E ratios versus volume-controlled ventilation on respiratory mechanics, gas exchange, and hemodynamics in patients with adult respiratory distress syndrome. Anesthesiology 1994;80:983–991.

PATIENT 29

A 25-week gestational age newborn girl with severe hypoxemia and respiratory distress

A 25-week gestational age girl developed severe respiratory distress immediately at birth. Of significance, she was born to an HIV-positive mother.

Physical Examination: Temperature 98.9°; pulse 140; respirations 40; blood pressure 100/60. Chest: bilateral breath sounds with poor chest excursion and diffuse rhonchi. Cardiac: tachycardia with no murmur. Abdomen: no bowel sounds, no masses, liver at costal margin. Extremities: cyanosis noted.

Laboratory Findings: WBC 16,000/μl, Hct 39.1%, platelets 65,000/μl. ABG (FiO$_2$ 1.0): pH 7.24, pCO$_2$ 69 mmHg, pO$_2$ 48 mmHg. Chest radiograph (see below): diffuse infiltrates.

Hospital Course: Artificial surfactant was administered and the patient was placed on mechanical ventilation. Despite this, adequate oxygenation could not be achieved. A consultation was requested for possible institution of extracorporeal membrane oxygenation (ECMO).

Questions: Which patients are likely to benefit from ECMO? What considerations are important before instituting ECMO?

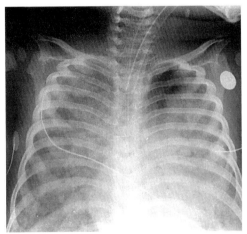 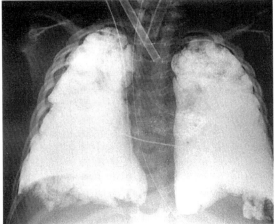

Diagnosis: Infant respiratory distress syndrome.

Discussion: Infant respiratory distress syndrome is caused by inadequate surfactant maturity and function associated with premature birth. The prognosis for this disorder has improved markedly in recent years with the development of exogenously administered surfactant. However, despite the use of this therapy, there still are infants in whom severe hypoxemia persists and additional therapeutic approaches are needed.

In the 1970s, **extracorporeal membrane oxygenation** (ECMO) was developed as a means of providing tissue oxygenation while bypassing severely damaged and essentially useless lungs. In recent years, ECMO has been combined with extracorporeal CO_2 removal ($ECCO_2R$) to help maintain a better acid–base balance. ECMO can be performed using a vein-to-artery (VA) approach, in a manner similar to the cardiopulmonary bypass used in open-heart surgery, or via a vein-to-vein (VV) mode, which is more commonly the approach when only respiratory assistance is the goal. In both approaches, blood is passed through a membrane bubble oxygenator and O_2 and CO_2 diffuse across a semipermeable membrane. The technical demands of the system are considerable, and may explain in part the infrequent use of this technique.

Clinical trials of ECMO have yielded conflicting results. The most recent large study of this technique in adult respiratory distress syndrome (ARDS) indicated no real survival benefit in patients treated with ECMO, and in the United States there is little enthusiasm for ECMO for ARDS. However, the technique is believed to offer a **survival advantage in neonatal and pediatric populations**. Though the VA technique has been the most widely employed, it requires access via the common carotid artery, and a reluctance to sacrifice this vessel has led to more widespread use of the VV approach, with partial ventilatory support.

There is a national registry of ECMO use which provides some data regarding outcome of neonates and children treated with the technique. For infants with meconium aspiration and the infant respiratory distress syndrome, registry survival has been 93% and 86%, respectively. In neonates with pneumonia, survival is slightly worse, at 77%. In the pediatric age group, survival after ECMO treatment of respiratory failure from a variety of causes, including bacterial and viral pneumonia, aspiration, and ARDS, has ranged from 29–67%. These data stand in contrast to results obtained in adults, where survival over 50% is uncommon; however, data on adult patients are minimal.

The many potential complications of ECMO fall into two major categories: hemorrhagic and mechanical. **Hemorrhagic complications** include intracerebral bleeding and bleeding at the operative site, while **mechanical problems** include clotting within the circuitry, malfunctions of the equipment, pump failure, and tubing rupture. Other side effects include renal dysfunction and hypotension. Because of these complications and the variable success rates reported with this supportive approach, ECMO-$ECCO_2R$ remains outside the standard respiratory armamentarium and only should be used in specific circumstances in centers with appropriately trained personnel.

The present patient, placed on ECMO-$ECCO_2R$, continued to demonstrate severe hypoxemia. Partial liquid ventilation was added, and the infant's respiratory status improved. Eventually she was weaned from the ventilator and discharged home.

Clinical Pearls

1. ECMO can be provided through a vein-to-artery approach or a vein-to-vein approach, with the latter method avoiding sacrifice of the common carotid artery.

2. Survival in patients treated with ECMO appears to be better in neonates and children than in adults, though this may be related more to underlying disease states than to the efficacy of this mode of support.

3. ECMO cannot be considered a standard mode of artificial respiratory support in either pediatric or adult populations.

REFERENCES

1. Paulson TE, Spear RM, Peterson BM. New concepts in the treatment of children with acute respiratory distress syndrome. J Pediatr 1995;127:163–175.
2. Plotkin JS, Shah JB, Lofland GK, DeWolf AM. Extracorporeal membrane oxygenation in the successful treatment of traumatic adult respiratory distress syndrome: Case report and review. J Trauma 1994;37:127–130.
3. Kanto WP Jr. A decade of experience with neonatal extracorporeal membrane oxygenation. J Pediatr 1994;124:335–347.
4. Morris AH, Wallace CJ, Menlove RL, et al. Randomized clinical trial of pressure-controlled inverse ratio ventilation and extracorporeal CO_2 removal for adult respiratory distress syndrome. Am J Respir Crit Care Med 1994;149:295–305.
5. Levy FH, O'Rourke PP, Crone RK. Extracorporeal membrane oxygenation. Anesth Analg 1992;75:1053–1062.

PATIENT 30

A full-term newborn infant girl with respiratory failure

A full-term infant girl was born after an uncomplicated pregnancy to a 34-year-old mother and was noted to have severe respiratory distress immediately at birth. Mechanical ventilation was immediately initiated.

Physical Examination: Temperature 98.6°; pulse 136; respirations 42, assisted; blood pressure 62/48; weight 3280 gm. Chest: breath sounds L > R with distant, diffuse rhonchi. Cardiac: no murmur. Head: anterior fontanel soft, endotracheal tube in place. Abdomen: soft, slightly scaphoid, umbilical lines in place. Extremities: cyanotic.

Laboratory Findings: ABG (FiO$_2$ 1.0): pH 7.34, pCO$_2$ 47 mmHg, pO$_2$ 28 mmHg. Chest radiograph: see below left.

Hospital Course: Upon delivery, the infant was transferred to the neonatal intensive care unit where she developed progressive respiratory failure, requiring high-frequency jet ventilation (HFJV) and veno-arterial extracorporeal membrane oxygenation (ECMO) at 2 hours of age.

Question: What is the diagnosis?

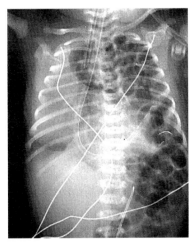 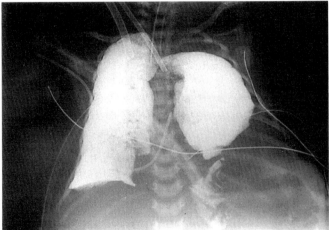

Diagnosis: Congenital diaphragmatic hernia resulting in pulmonary hypoplasia and respiratory failure.

Discussion: There are several congenital developmental disorders involving the diaphragm that have the potential to create severe respiratory distress in the newborn infant. These include congenital anterior diaphragmatic hernia (Morgagni's hernia), congenital diaphragmatic hernia of Bochdalek, congenital hiatal diaphragmatic hernia, and congenital eventration of the diaphragm. Of these, by far the most serious in terms of respiratory compromise is the **congenital diaphragmatic hernia of Bochdalek**, which is said to occur in one of 2200–3500 live births, accounting for 8% of major congenital anomalies.

Bochdalek's hernia results from a failure of closure of the pleuroperitoneal canal, which is developmentally the last portion of the diaphragm to close during gestation. The posterior portion of the diaphragm, the site of Bochdalek's hernia, usually closes in the 6th to 8th week of gestation, when the developing fetus is roughly 20 mm long. Eighty-five to 90% of Bochdalek's hernias occur on the left, as this side usually closes later.

The major consequence of Bochdalek's hernia is compression of the ipsilateral lung, with resultant **lack of lung development**. Alveolar buds develop days 75–90 of gestation, but the hernia usually is already present by the 48th day. Although the lung ipsilateral to the hernia is most directly affected, the contralateral lung usually suffers as well, because the mediastinal structures shift to that side. As a result of the compression of both fetal lungs, pulmonary hypoplasia and pulmonary vascular hypertension develop, both of which contribute to respiratory failure.

Diagnosis of a congenital diaphragmatic hernia is suggested whenever there is severe respiratory distress at birth. Plain chest radiographs are almost always diagnostic, displaying the typical findings (present in this case): a shifted mediastinum, very little aerated lung, nonvisualization of the diaphragm on the affected side, gas-filled bowel in the thorax, and an absence of gas-filled structures in the abdomen. The differential diagnosis, usually not difficult, includes multiple pulmonary pneumatocoeles, congenital cysts, cystic adenomatoid malformations, laryngotracheal obstruction, atelectasis, pneumothorax, phrenic nerve paralysis, and eventration.

Though treatment of Bochdalek's hernia ultimately is surgical, current practice involves an initial period of medical stabilization. Once the patient has stabilized, the hernia is closed via an abdominal approach if the repair is done early, or through a thoracic incision for later repairs. Major perioperative concerns include management of respiratory failure and pulmonary hypertension seen in these patients. A variety of approaches, including extracorporeal membrane oxygenation (ECMO) and partial liquid ventilation, have been tried.

Poor prognostic signs in the newborn period include the early onset of respiratory failure despite mechanical ventilatory intervention and the lack of a "honeymoon period" in which gas exchange is preserved for several hours to days after delivery. Additionally, a low functional residual capacity may be predictive of fatal pulmonary hyperplasia. Finally, the requirement for a diaphragmatic patch during repair, indicative of a large diaphragmatic defect, also is a poor prognostic sign. If pulmonary function does not improve and the patient cannot be weaned from ECMO, an aggressive approach to volume recruitment may be necessary. Bronchoscopy, to rule out structural and/or mechanical reasons for persistent atelectasis, treatment with steroids and exogenous surfactant, or, lastly, support with partial liquid ventilation (PLV) may be considered.

The present patient had perfluorochemical liquid instilled, while stable on ECMO therapy, to a level of 8 ml/kg within the first half-hour. By four hours, 30 ml/kg had been administered, suggesting considerable lung volume recruitment (see chest radiograph on previous page at right). Pulmonary compliance doubled, most likely due to the increased lung volume. PLV was continued for 96 hours with vigorous suctioning of debris and replacement of lost fluid. Despite significant improvements in pulmonary function, the infant succumbed to severe pulmonary hypertension on day 30 of life.

Clinical Pearls

1. Congenital diaphragmatic hernia is one of the most common causes of severe respiratory distress in newborns.

2. Congenital diaphragmatic hernia carries a poor prognosis in patients with severe pulmonary hyperplasia and persistence of pulmonary hypertension.

3. Treatment with partial liquid ventilation may be successful in volume recruitment and debris removal, but probably will not be sufficiently beneficial in helping infants with severe irreversible pulmonary hypertension.

REFERENCES

1. Antunes MJ, Greenspan JS, Cullen JA, et al. Prognosis with preoperative pulmonary function and lung volume assessment in infants with congenital diaphragmatic hernia. Pediatrics 1995;96:1117–1122.
2. Wilson JM, Lung DP, Lillehei CW, et al. Delayed repair and preoperative ECMO does not improve survival and high-risk congenital diaphragmatic hernia. J Pediatr Surg 1992;27:368–375.
3. Van Meurs KP, Newman KD, Anderson KD. Effective extracorporeal membrane oxygenation on survival of infants with congenital diaphragmatic hernia. J Pediatr 1990;117:954–960.
4. Bohn D, Tamura M, Perrin D, et al. Ventilator predictors of pulmonary hyperplasia in congenital diaphragmatic hernia, confirmed by morphologic assessment. J Pediatr 1987;11:423–431.

PATIENT 31

A 53-year-old man with hypercapneic respiratory failure and hypotension

A 53-year-old man with a history of asthma requiring only intermittent use of an albuterol metered-dose inhaler (MDI) was brought to the emergency department with a chief complaint of severe dypsnea.

Physical Examination: Temperature 98.9°; pulse 110; respirations 28; blood pressure 130/90, with a pulsus paradoxus of 18 mmHg. Chest: diffuse bilateral expiratory wheezing. Cor: regular rhythm, without murmurs. Abdomen: soft, without masses or organomegaly. Extremities: no cyanosis or clubbing. Neurologic: alert and oriented.

Laboratory Findings: ABG (40% ventimask): pH 7.45, pCO_2 33 mmHg, pO_2 130 mmHg, HCO_3^- 22 mEq/L, SaO_2 99%. Peak expiratory flow rate 160 lpm. Chest radiograph (see below): without infiltrates.

Hospital Course: The patient was given 60 mg of intravenous methylprednisolone and two sprays of albuterol via MDI every 20 minutes with a spacer. His condition deteriorated over the next 4 hours and he required intubation. Mechanical ventilation was initiated with a Bennett 7200 ventilator at the following settings: V_t 800 ml, f = 14 CMV, FiO_2 0.4, no PEEP. Repeat ABG: pH 7.30, pCO_2 54 mmHg, pO_2 123 mmHg, HCO_3^- 23 mEq/L, SaO_2 99%. The respiratory rate was increased to 20 bpm. Within 5 minutes, the blood pressure dropped to 80/50 and the pulse rate rose from 90 to 120 beats. Repeat ABG: pH 7.22, pCO_2 78 mmHg, pO_2 62 mmHg, HCO_3^- 24 mEq/L, SaO_2 94%.

Questions: What is the etiology of the patient's hypotension? What are the mechanical ventilatory considerations in the management of this patient?

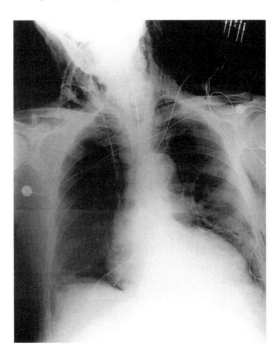

Diagnosis: Hemodynamic compromise secondary to the development of high level, intrinsic PEEP.

Discussion: Intrinsic PEEP (PEEP$_i$), also called auto-PEEP or dynamic hyperinflation (DHI), is the phenomenon of **positive end-expiratory pressure** at the alveolar level secondary to end-expiratory gas trapping at volumes greater than the functional residual capacity. It is usually produced unintentionally, is often occult, and may result in significant morbidity and mortality. PEEP$_i$ in a mechanically ventilated patient results from the triggering of a positive pressure breath prior to complete exhalation of the previous breath. Auto-PEEP develops when the ventilator delivers a new breath before the previous exhalation has been completed, resulting in hyperinflation. Thus, PEEP$_i$ is promoted by factors that impede full exhalation of tidal volume. These include airway obstruction, secretions, inflammatory mucosa, and dynamic closure of small airways during exhalation. PEEP$_i$ also may develop in those mechanically ventilated patients who require large minute ventilations with short expiratory times and high inspiration/expiration (I:E) ratios.

PEEP$_i$ may be transmitted to the pleural space, causing a reduction in transmural central venous pressure and decreasing venous return and cardiac output. This results in tachycardia, hypotension, or obstructive shock. DHI, especially in chronic lung patients with normal or elevated static compliance, can lead to alveolar overdistention with resultant barotrauma or volutrauma.

PEEP$_i$ increases the work of breathing in the following way: to trigger inspiratory flow through the demand valve of a ventilator in the IMV, CPAP, or PSV modes, the patient must exert a transpulmonary pressure gradient, lowering alveolar pressure below zero (or the PEEP level). This process normally requires only minimal effort with the assumption that a high sensitivity is set and the demand valve is "responsive." To initiate inspiration in the presence of auto-PEEP, patients must increase their efforts to lower intrapleural pressures by an amount equivalent to the PEEP$_i$. For this reason, some advocate that the best way to reduce excess work of breathing related to auto-PEEP is to set the ventilator PEEP to equal the measured auto-PEEP. Raising the ventilator driving pressure to the level of PEEP$_i$ facilitates patient-triggered inspiration because alveolar pressure only has to be reduced below the level of PEEP (to PEEP$_i$) to initiate a mechanical breath.

Trapped alveolar gas causing PEEP$_i$ is not displayed on the manometer during the normal respiratory cycle because the expiratory limb of the ventilator is open to the atmosphere. Unless suspected and reduced, significant levels of PEEP$_i$ may be overlooked as a common cause of problems in ventilated patients. These problems include agitation, pressure limiting of delivered tidal volumes, or more serious hemodynamic effects such as hypotension or electromechanical dissociation. If overlooked when interpreting hemodynamic variables, elevated levels of PEEP$_i$ can lead to erroneous decision making (transient elevations in pulmonary artery pressures).

Measuring auto-PEEP is relatively easy in the heavily sedated or paralyzed patient. Pausing the ventilatory cycle and occluding expiratory flow just prior to the next inspiration will allow equilibrium of the pressure within the system and PEEP$_i$ will be displayed on the manometer. Depending on the type of ventilator, expiratory flow can be stopped by crimping the tubing leading to the expiratory port, manually blocking the port, or pressing the "expiratory pause hold." In patients with no inspiratory effort, changes in airway pressure necessary to initiate flow should be PEEP$_i$ and can be measured. In patients who are making respiratory efforts, these estimations of auto-PEEP may be inaccurate.

PEEP$_i$ can be decreased or prevented by maximizing either the rate or time allowed for lung emptying. Strategies include use of large-bore endotracheal tubes and bronchodilators, and suctioning of airway secretions. The I:E ratio can be lowered by decreasing the respiratory rate or tidal volume, or by increasing the inspiratory flow rate.

The present patient was admitted with significant expiratory air flow obstruction due to a severe asthma attack. His condition deteriorated despite pharmacologic interventions. After intubation, he developed respiratory acidosis and hypotension. After PEEP$_i$ was detected, maneuvers were employed to decrease the minute volume and allow adequate expiratory time. The patient responded to this ventilatory course and was successfully weaned to extubation.

Clinical Pearls

1. Mechanically ventilated patients requiring large minute volumes or with inadequate expiratory times are at high risk for developing intrinsic PEEP.

2. Intrinsic PEEP may be transmitted to the pleural space, increasing the mean intrathoracic pressure, reducing venous return, dropping cardiac output, and producing hypotension.

3. Maneuvers that may be helpful in reducing or eliminating intrinsic PEEP include decreasing minute volume or increasing inspiratory flow rate.

REFERENCES

1. Leatherman JW, Ravenscraft SA. Low measured, auto-positive, end-expiratory pressure during mechanical ventilation of patients with severe asthma: Hidden auto-positive, end-expiratory pressure. Crit Care Med 1996;24:541–546.
2. Stewart TE, Slutsky AS. Occult, occult auto-PEEP in status asthmaticus. Crit Care Med 1996;24:379–380.
3. Baigorri F, de Monte A, Blanch L, et al. Hemodynamic responses to external counterbalancing of auto-positive, end-expiratory pressure in mechanically ventilated patients with chronic obstructive pulmonary disease. Crit Care Med 1994;22:1782–1791.
4. Tokioka H, Saito S, Saeki S, et al. The effect of pressure-support ventilation on auto-PEEP in a patient with asthma. Chest 1992;101:285–286.
5. Hoffman RA, Ershowsky P, Krieger B. Determination of auto-PEEP during spontaneous and controlled ventilation by monitoring changes in end-expiratory thoracic gas volume. Chest 1989;96:613–616.

PATIENT 32

**A 60-year-old man with unilateral loss of breath sounds and increased
A-a oxygen gradient following abdominal surgery**

A 60-year-old man was transferred to the recovery room following an uneventful left nephrectomy. On 50% oxygen, an intraoperative ABG had revealed a PaO_2 of 230 mmHg. After surgery, on 50% oxygen, the SaO_2 was 91%.

Physical Examination: Temperature 98°; pulse 90; respirations 14; blood pressure 136/92. Chest: markedly decreased breath sounds on the left. Endotracheal tube in place, taped at 20 cm, unchanged from its intraoperative position. Cardiac: normal. Abdomen: decreased bowel sounds. Extremities: no cyanosis. Neurologic: lethargic, but nonfocal.

Laboratory Findings: ABG (FiO_2 1.0): pH 7.39, pCO_2 38 mmHg, pO_2 67 mmHg, HCO_3^- 23 mEq/L, SaO_2 93%. Peak airway pressure 30 cm H_2O. Chest radiograph: see below.

Hospital Course: The patient was provided with aggressive pulmonary toilet with no change in the measured saturation. Peak airway pressures were high (55–60 cm H_2O), hypoxemia was refractory to an FiO_2 of 1.0, and markedly decreased breath sounds over the left hemithorax were again noted. Repeat chest radiography and an urgent fiberoptic bronchoscopy were performed.

Questions: What are the most likely etiologies of a unilateral decrease in breath sounds in a postoperative patient? What treatment options exist for this patient?

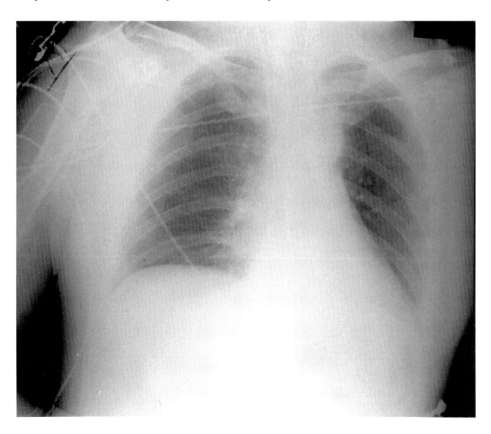

Diagnosis: Postoperative atelectasis due to a mucus plug occluding the left lower lobe bronchus.

Discussion: Pulmonary complications are the leading cause of postoperative morbidity and mortality. Atelectasis and pneumonia, the two most common pulmonary complications, are often related. Their frequencies vary with different types of surgery—cardiac, thoracic, and upper abdominal surgery place patients at greatest risk. Mechanical ventilation in any setting may be associated with segmental or lobar atelectasis. Acute collapse of large pulmonary segments, lobes, or an entire lung can produce acute respiratory failure by increasing the work of breathing as total compliance fails. In the intubated patient receiving mechanical ventilatory support, severe hypoxemia due to ventilation-perfusion mismatch and right-to-left intrapulmonary shunting may result. If left untreated, pneumonia can occur.

The most common cause of acute lobar collapse in the postoperative, intubated patient is **central airway occlusion** by mucus plugging and subsequent distal absorptive atelectasis. Additional causes include foreign body aspiration, multiple mucus plugs in smaller distal airways, and extensive regional microatelectasis without airway obstruction. In the postoperative patient requiring mechanical ventilatory support, decreased secretion clearance can occur for a number of reasons. Coughing is less effective or absent due to reduced vital capacity, supine position, pain, analgesia, sedation, and the presence of the endotracheal tube. Prolonged lobar dependence, decreased ciliary transport, abnormal mucus flow, and dehydration of secretions secondary to anesthesia may lead to stasis and subsequent airway obstruction. In addition, acute lobar collapse involving the left lower lobe remains a common problem in these patients despite efforts to increase bronchopulmonary toilet. This is because suctioning with standard catheters is more likely to remove secretions from the right main bronchus, due to the normal anatomic relationships of the main bronchi to the trachea. The newer catheters designed for left-sided suctioning may help with this problem.

Standard techniques of pulmonary hygiene and chest physiotherapy include frequent repositioning, postural drainage, percussion and vibration, and endotracheal suctioning. When significant atelectasis does occur, the optimal treatment depends on the clinical situation. Unless severe hypoxemia or refractoriness to treatment exists, the standard treatment for lobar collapse is **aggressive respiratory care**. In the mechanically ventilated patient, this includes chest physiotherapy, hyperexpansion with increased tidal volumes and PEEP, and increased tracheobronchial toilet using nebulized bronchodilators. For *preventing* postoperative complications, however, routine chest physiotherapy, including chest percussion, has not been shown to be advantageous when compared to early ambulation and the use of an incentive spirometer. In addition, the routine use of mucolytic therapy (n-acetylcysteine) administered as a nebulized solution is to be discouraged, as there is no good evidence that mucus plugs can be dissolved in this manner, and the substance can be quite irritating to the airways, resulting in worse bronchospasm.

In general, these measures are successful. If they are not, **fiberoptic bronchoscopy** (FOB) with direct visualization of the airways and directed secretion removal is the traditional alternative intervention. However, despite the likely role of secretions and mucus plugging in the initiation of lobar atelectasis, a mucus plug is found by FOB in only 41% of cases, and there is no indication for routine use of FOB to guide endotracheal suctioning in postoperative, intubated patients without mucus plugging and lobar collapse.

The present patient's recovery room chest radiograph revealed a left, lower lobar atelectasis which, when combined with the other clinical symptoms, prompted FOB. An obstructing plug was removed with subsequent rapid clinical improvement. The remaining recovery process was unremarkable, and the patient was extubated without difficulty.

Clinical Pearls

1. The differential diagnosis of unilateral absence of breath sounds in a mechanically ventilated patient includes pneumothorax and bronchial obstruction.

2. The left lower lobe is the area of the lung that most commonly becomes atelectatic.

3. The presence of an air bronchogram entering the atelectatic region on the chest radiograph predicts a poor response to treatment with standard therapy or fiberoptic bronchoscopy.

REFERENCES

1. Hall JC, Tarala RA, Hall JL. A case–control study of postoperative pulmonary complications after laparoscopic and open cholecystectomy. J Laparoendosc Surg 1996;6:87–92.
2. Johnson D, Kelm C, Thomson D, et al. The effect of physical therapy on respiratory complications following cardiac valve surgery. Chest 1996;109:638–644.
3. Joyce CJ, Baker AB. What is the role of absorption atelectasis in the genesis of perioperative pulmonary collapse? Anaesth Intensive Care 1995;23:691–696.
4. Kacmarek RM. Prophylactic bronchial hygiene following cardiac surgery: What is necessary? Intens Care Med 1995;21:467–468.
5. Johnson D, Kelm C, To T, et al. Postoperative physical therapy after coronary bypass surgery. Am J Resp Crit Care Med 1995;152:953–958.
6. Panacek EA, Albertson TE, Rutherford WF. Selective left endobronchial suctioning in the intubated patient. Chest 1989;95:885–887.

PATIENT 33

A 59-year-old man status post cardiac arrest and dependent on a ventilator for 2 months

A 59-year-old man was admitted to the ventilator-dependent unit of a long-term care facility. One month prior to admission, he sustained a cardiac arrest with a prolonged resuscitation effort in an acute care hospital where he had been admitted for pneumonia, hypertension, and coronary artery disease.

Physical Examination: Temperature 99°; pulse 80; respirations 16 and assisted; blood pressure 140/90. Chest: scattered rhonchi throughout. Tracheostomy tube in place. Cardiac: regular rhythm, without murmurs. Abdomen: without masses or organomegaly. Extremities: no cyanosis, clubbing, or edema. Neurologic: unresponsive, with pupils fixed and nonreactive to light.

Laboratory Findings: ABG (FiO$_2$ 0.3): pH 7.44, pCO$_2$ 110 mmHg, HCO$_3^-$ 28 mEq/L, SaO$_2$ 98%. Chest radiograph (see below): blunting of the left costophrenic angle and cardiomegaly.

Questions: What condition most likely explains the patient's clinical presentation? What are the general considerations in the care of this patient?

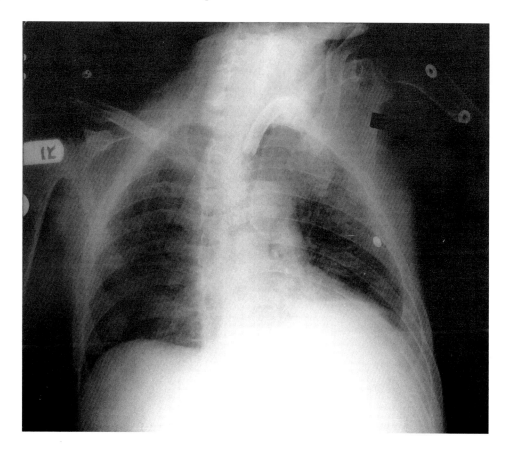

Diagnosis: Anoxic encephalopathy due to cardiac arrest.

Discussion: Anoxic encephalopathy is a common and often devastating condition caused by lack of oxygen to the brain as a result of hypotension or respiratory failure. Conditions that most often lead to anoxic encephalopathy include cardiac arrest, severe hemorrhage, suffocation, and carbon monoxide poisoning.

When severe hypoxia or anoxia occurs, as in cardiac arrest, consciousness is lost within seconds. Evidence of the event may include reduced oxygenation of arterial blood with a $PaO_2 < 40$ mmHg, carbon monoxide intoxication, blood pressures < 70 mmHg systolic, or cardiac arrest. Recovery can be complete if breathing, oxygenation of blood, and cardiac status is restored within 3–5 minutes. The diagnosis of anoxic encephalopathy depends on the history of a specific **hypoxic-ischemic event**. If anoxia persists beyond this time, there is often serious and permanent injury to the brain, particularly in those regions in which the efficiency of circulation is marginal. It is difficult to assess the precise degree of hypoxia-ischemia on a clinical basis, since even an imperceptible blood pressure may serve to maintain circulation to some extent. Hence, some individuals have made an excellent recovery after cerebral anoxia that reportedly lasted 8–10 minutes or longer; in general, however, prolonged resuscitation efforts are more likely to be associated with a poor neurologic outcome.

Extreme or sustained global ischemia results in **brain death**. Immediately following resuscitation from cardiopulmonary arrest, the physical findings may suggest brain death. These findings include dilated, unresponsive pupils; absent brainstem reflexes and respiration; and isoelectric electroencephalography traces. In many states in the U.S., brain death is now legally equated with death, but neurologic findings of brain death must be present and stable for many hours in cases of nontraumatic brain injury before such a determination can be made. Though a variety of diagnostic modalities

have been studied for their abilities to predict neurologic recovery after anoxic injury, it has been convincingly shown that when the unresponsive state persists for more than a few hours, the prognosis is poor. Thus, patients with nontraumatic brain injury and severe deficits persisting for more than 24 hours are unlikely to have significant recovery.

Following resuscitation, neurologic evaluation typically reveals a patient who is profoundly comatose, with divergent, motionless eyes but reactive pupils. Limbs may be flaccid or intensely rigid and tendon reflexes are diminished. Generalized convulsions, muscle twitches (myoclonus), decerebrate or decorticate postures, and Babinski signs may all be present or evoked. The individual may survive in an irreversible **coma**, sometimes referred to as a persistent vegetative state. These patients remain mute, unresponsive, and unaware of their environments. Patients in deep coma lasting more than a few days rarely experience a full recovery.

Patients with lesser degrees of injury improve after a period of coma. Consciousness is regained and varying degrees of confusion, mind blindness, extrapyramidal rigidity, or movement disorder become evident. Some of these patients pass quickly through the post-hypoxic phase and make a full recovery; others are left with permanent neurologic sequelae.

The treatment of anoxic encephalopathy is directed primarily at the prevention of a critical degree of hypoxic injury. Following the establishment of a clear and secure airway, measures such as artifical respiration, external cardiac massage, the use of a cardiac defibrillator and/or pacemaker, and open chest surgery all have a place. Prompt resuscitation is critical, and in the setting of unwitnessed cardiac arrest, both in- and out-of-hospital resuscitative efforts are unlikely to be of much benefit.

The patient persists in a vegetative state requiring ventilatory support and total nursing care in a sub-acute nursing facility.

Clinical Pearls

1. Degrees of hypoxia that at no time abolish consciousness rarely cause permanent damage to the central nervous system.

2. The duration of cardiac arrest before resuscitation efforts have begun is correlated with survival and neurologic outcome.

3. Electroencephalography is a good neurologic indicator of patient prognosis following cardiopulmonary resuscitation.

4. Neurologic recovery is indirectly proportional to the amount of time a patient spends in an unresponsive state.

REFERENCES

1. Cobbe SM, Dalziel K, Ford I, Marsden AK. Survival of 1476 patients initially resuscitated from out of hospital cardiac arrest. BMJ 1996;312:1633–1637.
2. Yamashita S, Morinaga T, Ohgo S. Prognostic value of electroencephalogram (EEG) in anoxic encephalopathy after cardiopulmonary resuscitation: Relationship among anoxic period, EEG grading and outcome. Intern Med 1995;34:71–76.
3. Berek K, Lechleitner P, Luef G, et al. Early determination of neurological outcome after prehospital cardiopulmonary resuscitation. Stroke 1995;26:543–549.
4. Bialecki L, Woodward RS. Predicting death after CPR. Experience at a nonteaching community hospital with a full-time critical care staff. Chest 1995;108:1009–1017.
5. Levy DE, Caronna JJ, Singer BH, et al. Predicting outcome from hypoxic-ischemic coma. JAMA 1985;253: 1420–1426.

PATIENT 34

A 34-year-old man with dizziness and an unsteady gait for 2 weeks

A 34-year-old man was brought to the emergency department complaining of dizziness and an unsteady gait for 2 weeks. He had a history of a seizure disorder secondary to head trauma, and 2 weeks prior to admission he had experienced increased seizure activity, at which point his phenytoin was increased from 200 mg to 300 mg bid. Phenytoin levels were drawn and the patient returned home. Current medications included phenytoin, carbamazepine, and folic acid. The patient was allergic to penicillin.

Physical Examination: Temperature 98.1°; pulse 78; respirations 18; blood pressure 130/80. HEENT: cervical lymphadenopathy. Chest: normal. Cardiac: regular rhythm, without murmurs. Abdomen: without masses or organomegaly. Extremities: no cyanosis or clubbing. Neurologic: lethargic; lateral gaze nystagmus present, otherwise nonfocal exam.

Laboratory Findings: Glucose 62 mg/dl. CBC, liver function tests: normal. Pulse oximetry (nasal cannula O_2 2 L/min): 96%. Phenytoin 52.7 µg/ml, carbamazepine 4.7 µg/ml. EKG: normal sinus rhythm without ST-T wave abnormalities. Chest radiograph: see below.

Questions: What is the most likely cause of the patient's symptoms? What is the general approach to the care of this patient?

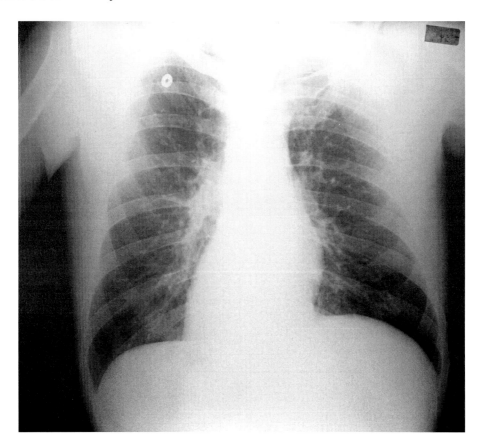

Diagnosis: Phenytoin toxicity.

Discussion: The treatment of patients with seizure disorders is directed at eliminating the cause and suppressing the expression. The fundamental modality for the treatment of epilepsy is pharmacologic therapy, and the overall goal is to protect the patient from having seizures without affecting normal cognitive function. Therefore, it is important that the patient be treated with the lowest possible dose of a single antiepileptic medication that avoids producing harmful systemic side effects. Precise knowledge of the kind of seizure the patient is having and the spectrums of action and pharmacokinetic principles of available antiepileptics can result in complete control of seizures in many patients.

Phenytoin (diphenylhydantoin, Dilantin) is a mainstay in the treatment of seizure disorders, and it is commonly used both for tonic-clonic and partial seizure activity. It is believed to work by stabilizing cell membranes through (blocking) action on sodium channels and calcium uptake during depolarization and by causing an increase in Na-K ATPase activity and Cl⁻ conductance. Phenytoin carries an average half-life of 10–15 hours when given intravenously and 22 hours when taken orally. For the chronic management of patients with seizure disorders, the therapeutic blood level of the drug is 10–20 µg/ml, and 90% of the drug is protein-bound. Because of these electrophysiologic effects, disturbances in cardiac conduction may occur.

Though serum levels are available to guide management, many patients will develop **side effects** related to phenytoin use, even at therapeutic drug levels. These side effects include ataxia, nausea, vomiting, rash, fever, hepatitis, sedation, and confusion. The devastating Stevens-Johnson syndrome has been reported, but only rarely. Fortunately, most of the side effects are uncommon and can be predicted from blood levels. Dizziness usually occurs at levels > 30 µg/ml and lethargy at levels > 40 µg/ml. With chronic administration, gingival hyperplasia and pseudolymphoma may also occur.

There is little evidence that phenytoin has direct effects on the respiratory system, and depression of ventilatory drive is generally not a feature of phenytoin use or overdose, though coma may occur at extremely high levels. However, an interesting but probably rare respiratory complication of phenytoin use recently has been reported. A child receiving phenytoin was noted to have frequent respiratory infections and deficiency of both IgG2 and IgG4 production. When phenytoin administration was stopped, the IgG subclass levels returned to normal and the child no longer had respiratory infections.

Rarely, phenytoin administration has been reported to cause a pneumonitis, manifested by shortness of breath, abnormal chest radiograph, and a positive [67]gallium citrate scan showing increased uptake in the lungs. These symptoms resolve after the drug is withdrawn.

Of the many **drug interactions** which occur with phenytoin, one is of particular interest in the care of pulmonary patients. Patients receiving antituberculous (anti-TB) chemotherapy, especially with isoniazid, are at risk for phenytoin toxicity because of the effect of anti-TB medications on hepatic metabolism of the anticonvulsant. For this reason, anticonvulsant drug levels should be closely monitored in patients receiving both phenytoin and anti-TB therapy.

The treatment of phenytoin overdose or toxicity is generally supportive, and withdrawal of the drug is, of course, the mainstay of therapy. The present patient underwent a complete analysis of critical blood chemistries, including liver function tests. Fortunately, despite the significantly elevated blood level of phenytoin, no dangerous cardiopulmonary or neurologic compromise was noted. He was discharged from the hospital 3 days after admission.

Clinical Pearls

1. Phenytoin, a commonly used antiepileptic, is associated with a wide range of common side effects, including nystagmus (seen at therapeutic levels) and ataxia (a sign of toxicity).

2. Respiratory complications of phenytoin use are uncommon, though pneumonitis has been reported, as has a decrease in IgG production leading to respiratory infection.

3. A drug interaction with isoniazid occurs commonly with phenytoin administration, leading to increased anticonvulsant levels. Phenytoin levels should be followed closely in patients receiving these two drugs together.

REFERENCES

1. Walubo A, Aboo A. Phenytoin toxicity due to concomitant antituberculosis therapy. Afr Med J 1995;85:1175–1176.
2. Khan AS, Dadparvar S, Brown SJ, et al. The role of gallium-67-citrate in the detection of phenytoin-induced pneumonitis. J Nucl Med 1994;35:471–473.
3. Ishizaka A, Nakanishi M, Kasahara E, et al. Phenytoin-induced IgG2 and IgG4 deficiencies in a patient with epilepsy. Acta Paediatr 1992;81:646–648.
4. Harris DW, Ostlere L, Buckley C, et al. Phenytoin-induced pseudolymphoma. A report of a case and review of the literature. Brit J Dermatol 1992;127:403–406.

PATIENT 35

**A 53-year-old man with multiple fractures after being struck
by a fast-moving car**

A 53-year-old man was crossing the street when he was struck by a motor vehicle travelling at a high rate of speed. While on the ground, he was struck by a second vehicle and received multiple fractures.

Physical Examination: Temperature 97.7°; pulse 120; respirations 20; blood pressure 96/palpation. HEENT: bilateral periorbital ecchymoses (raccoon eyes), epistaxis, right supraorbital laceration. Chest: bilateral, equal breath sounds; trachea midline. Cardiac: regular rhythm, without murmurs. Abdomen: rigid and tender to palpation. Extremities: no cyanosis. Neurologic: confused, but without gross focal findings.

Laboratory Findings: WBC 22,900/μl, Hct 30.2%. O_2 saturation: 86% by pulse oximetry. Chest radiograph: see below.

Hospital Course: The patient was brought to the emergency department with two intravenous lines of lactated Ringers solution running wide and with MAST pants on and fully inflated. He was intubated and placed on a Siemens Servo 900C ventilator with the following settings: volume control mode, V_t 900 ml, f = 16, FiO_2 1.0.

Question: What is the most likely explanation for the patient's hypotension and anemia?

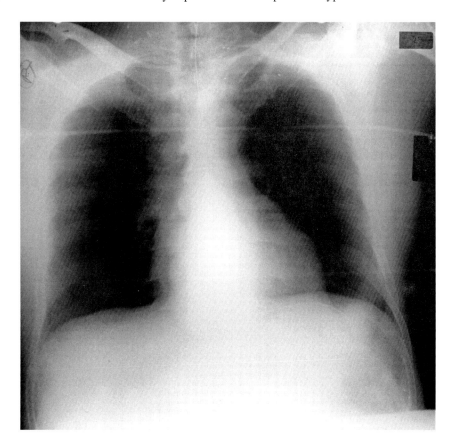

Answer: Hypovolemic shock due to splenic tear and hepatic rupture.

Discussion: Shock is an acute clinical syndrome initiated by systemic hypoperfusion and should be considered a **continuum of pathologic alterations** that become progressively more severe. The primary defect underlying all forms of acute circulatory failure (shock) is reduction of effective blood flow with inadequate tissue perfusion and a decrease in the delivery of oxygen to the capillary exchange bed. In the face of inadequate perfusion, lactic acid accumulates as a result of anaerobic glycolysis; measurement of this accumulation allows an estimate of the perfusion failure and the oxygen deficit.

Shock can be classified into four types of circulatory abnormalities: hypovolemic, cardiogenic, distributive, and septic. Hypovolemic shock is the condition in which the volume within the intravascular compartment is inadequate for tissue perfusion. Hemorrhage or a large loss of fluid secondary to trauma, vomiting, diarrhea, burns, or dehydration leads to inadequate ventricular filling. There is a markedly reduced preload, reflected by decreased left and right ventricular end-diastolic volumes and pressures. These changes lead to shock by causing an inadequate stroke volume and subsequent diminished cardiac output. Hypovolemic shock is classified as Stage I, 15% intravascular volume loss; Stage II, 20–25% intravascular volume loss; Stage III, 30–35% intravascular volume loss and the development of progressive signs and symptoms of shock; and Stage IV, more than 40% intravascular volume loss and unresponsiveness with an approximate 90% mortality.

The human body is rich with compensatory mechanisms aimed at reducing persistent inadequate tissue perfusion. In hypovolemia, one of the earliest compensatory mechanisms is **peripheral vasoconstriction** to create peripheral shunting that redistributes perfusion from the periphery to the central thorax. In addition to fluid shifting from the interstitial to the intravascular compartments, increased heart rate and inotropy are appreciated in hypovolemia.

Shortly after hemorrhagic trauma, stimulation of sympathetic and adrenal medullary activity begins, resulting in vasoconstriction that increases peripheral vascular resistance and maintains blood pressure. Increases in heart rate and stroke volume are also aimed at increasing cardiac output and maintaining blood pressure and organ perfusion.

Shock is almost always characterized by **hypotension**. In adults, this generally refers to a mean arterial pressure of less than 60 mmHg. Other manifestations include tachycardia; oliguria; altered mentation; and cool, mottled extremities indicative of reduced blood flow to the skin. Metabolic acidosis, due to elevated blood lactic acid levels, reflects prolonged inadequate blood flow to multiple tissues.

Management of the patient with shock begins during resuscitation and does not end until all bodily tissues are being properly perfused. Therapy must be instituted as quickly as possible to prevent permanent end-organ damage. Placement of large-bore intravenous lines for transfusion of blood and fluid resuscitation are imperative as initial measures. At the same time, a complete clinical assessment must be made rapidly to ensure a thorough understanding of the cause of the condition. A history is taken immediately, and a physical examination as well as specific diagnostic procedures directed towards determining the cause and severity of the condition are performed.

Most patients with fully developed shock require tracheal intubation and mechanical ventilatory support, even if acute respiratory failure, as seen with arterial blood gases, is not yet present. These measures are required to protect the airway and to reduce the work of breathing in patients whose oxygen delivery may be marginal. Hypoxemia refractory to supplemental oxygen therapy mandates mechanical ventilatory support. Endotracheal intubation is indicated if changes in mentation make protection of the airway uncertain or when inadequate compensation for a metabolic acidosis is life-threatening.

The present patient was stabilized during a brief stay in the emergency room and then taken directly to the operating room where on laparotomy he was found to have a severely lacerated liver and spleen. The blood loss could not be stemmed, and he succumbed to his injuries.

Clinical Pearls

1. Perfusion of the coronary and cerebral vessels is maintained at a mean arterial pressure above 70 mmHg.

2. In hypovolemia, initial vasoconstriction maintains blood pressure; however, after a loss of approximately 25–33% of the intravascular volume, hypotension develops.

3. Oxygen therapy is indicated in all cases of hypovolemia shock as inadequate tissue perfusion leads to anaerobic glycolysis with concomitant lactacidemia and hypoxemia.

REFERENCES

1. Cutress R. Fluid resuscitation in traumatic haemorrhage. J Accid Emerg Med 1995;12:165–172.
2. Pollack CV Jr. Prehospital fluid resuscitation of the trauma patient. An update on the controversies. Emerg Med Clin North Am 1993;11:61–70.
3. Cooper C, Militello P. The multi-injured patient: The Maryland shock trauma protocol approach. Semin Thorac Cardiovasc Surg 1992;4:163–167.
4. Trunkey D. Initial treatment of patients with extensive trauma. New Engl J Med 1991;324:1259–1263.

PATIENT 36

A 32-year-old woman with unresponsiveness and seizures

A 32-year-old woman with a history of a seizure disorder and systemic lupus erythematosus was brought to the emergency department with unresponsiveness following a seizure that occurred after a 3-day course of fever, chills, and general lethargy. She was intubated on arrival.

Physical Examination: Temperature 100.9°; pulse 110; respirations assisted; blood pressure 90/60. Chest: rhonchi throughout. Cardiac: regular rhythm, without murmurs. Abdomen: soft, liver edge palpable 3 fingerbreadths below the costal margin. Extremities: no cyanosis or clubbing. Neurologic: unresponsive, with reactive pupils.

Laboratory Findings: WBC 15,500/µl, Hct 36.7%. Chloride 126 mEq/L, BUN 47 mg/dl, Cr 3.6 mg/dl. PT 27.2 sec, PTT 120 sec, control 12.1 sec. Aspartate aminotransferase 945 IU/L, alanine aminotransferase 118 IU/L, amylase 737 IU/L. Antinuclear antibodies positive, 1:160. ABG (FiO$_2$ 1.0): pH 7.49, pCO$_2$ 36 mmHg, pO$_2$ 76 mmHg, HCO$_3^-$ 28 mEq/L, SaO$_2$ 96%. A pulmonary artery catheter was placed and yielded the following readings: cardiac output 6.5 L/min, PAS/PAD 32/20 mmHg, pulmonary artery occlusion pressure (wedge pressure) 18–20 mmHg. Chest radiograph (see below): bibasilar infiltrates.

Question: What are the reasons for this patient's gas exchange and radiographic abnormalities?

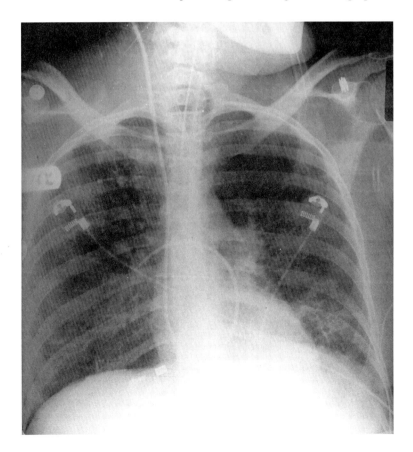

Diagnosis: Pneumonia and early adult respiratory distress syndrome in a patient with systemic lupus erythematosus.

Discussion: Systemic lupus erythematosus (SLE) is a multisystem disease characterized by the deposition of complement proteins and immunoglobulins in tissues with a marked inflammatory response. The cause of lupus is unknown, though the disease is marked by the presence of circulating antibodies against the body's own antigens, such as antinuclear antibodies and antibodies against double-stranded DNA. There is a predominance of women (particularly African-Americans) among patients with lupus, and the age range for disease onset is 15–25. Typical early manifestations of the disease include the characteristic butterfly (malar) rash on the face, joint pains, oral ulcers, renal dysfunction, pericarditis, and pleuritis. Central nervous system involvement, manifest by seizures and mental status changes, may also occur. Treatment of lupus is with immunosuppressive therapy, beginning with corticosteroids but often requiring more powerful agents such as azathioprine.

Pulmonary involvement in lupus can take several forms. The most common thoracic manifestation of SLE is **pleuritis**, characterized by an inflammatory pleural effusion without parenchymal involvement. The fluid typically has a high protein level and the cellular response may be characterized by the presence of LE cells, which are specific for the diagnosis. Pleurisy generally responds to treatment with nonsteroidal anti-inflammatory agents or prednisone.

Pulmonary **infections** are a major lung complication in patients with lupus, and the occurrence of bacterial pneumonia and other infections is related both to the SLE itself, with its underlying derangements of the immune system, and to the immunosuppressive therapy used to treat the disease. Thus, although common pathogens such as *S. pneumoniae* and *H. influenzae* are seen in lupus patients, diseases such as *Pneumocystis carinii* pneumonia have been reported in SLE patients receiving corticosteroids and should be in the differential diagnosis. Tuberculosis and fungal diseases should also be considered potential pathogens in this setting.

Acute lupus pneumonitis, although not uncommon, is a poorly characterized pathological entity. Patients with this syndrome usually are quite ill, and they present with fever, hypoxia, and pulmonary infiltrates in the absence of an identifiable infectious agent. Therapy consists of high-dose immunosuppressive therapy to which antibiotics generally are added. As infectious complications of lupus outnumber cases of acute lupus pneumonitis by a large margin, it is important to retain antibiotic therapy when treating patients with this syndrome. A similar strategy is employed in another pulmonary complication of lupus, the alveolar hemorrhage syndrome, in which bleeding is a result of the vasculitis that occurs in the alveolar-capillary unit. It is important to remember that not all patients with alveolar hemorrhage have obvious hemoptysis.

Pulmonary **embolism** may also complicate SLE, often in patients with the anticardiolipin antibody syndrome (one of the antiphospholipid antibodies or circulating lupus anticoagulants). Chronic pulmonary complications of SLE include pulmonary **hypertension**, pulmonary **fibrosis**, and the so-called shrinking lung syndrome, in which lung volumes progressively diminish, perhaps because of diaphragmatic weakness. This latter disorder can be difficult to distinguish from restrictive lung disease associated with early fibrosis.

The current patient's hypoxemia and early infiltrates were suggestive of the acute pneumonitis syndrome. Despite glucocorticoids, broad spectrum antibiotics, and hemodynamic support, she developed septic shock complicated by the hepatorenal syndrome and expired 4 days after admission.

Clinical Pearls

1. Systemic lupus erythematosus is a multisystem disease characterized by repeated episodes of inflammation in the kidneys, skin, lungs, and other organs.

2. Acute pulmonary complications of lupus include bacterial and opportunistic infections, acute pneumonitis, alveolar hemorrhage, and pulmonary embolism.

3. Patients with acute lupus pneumonitis generally should receive antibiotics along with immunosuppression, as infections can be difficult to exclude from this syndrome on clinical grounds.

REFERENCES

1. Foster HE, Malleson PN, Petty RE, et al. *Pneumocystis carinii* pneumonia in childhood systemic lupus erythematosus. J Rheumatol 1996;23:753–756.
2. Orens JB, Martinez FJ, Lynch JP 3rd. Pleuropulmonary manifestations of systemic lupus erythematosus. Rheum Dis Clin N Am 1994;20:159–193.
3. Schwab EP, Schumacher HR Jr, Freundlich B, Callegari PE. Pulmonary alveolar hemorrhage in systemic lupus erythematosus. Semin Arthritis Rheum 1993;23:8–15.
4. Porges AJ, Beattie SL, Ritchlin C, et al. Patients with systemic lupus erythematosus at risk for *Pneumocystis carinii* pneumonia. J Rheumatol 1992;19:1191–1194.

PATIENT 37

A 26-day-old infant boy with a dry cough, runny nose, and fever for 2 days

A 26-day-old infant boy was brought to the emergency department with a dry cough and fever. He had been sick for 2 days. The mother's pregnancy and delivery had been uncomplicated.

Physical Examination: Temperature 101.6°; pulse 174; respirations 72 with substernal retractions; blood pressure 102/82. HEENT: hyperemic pharynx, rhinorrhea, and a normal inner ear. Chest: expiratory wheezing throughout. Cardiac: tachycardic, without murmurs. Abdomen: soft, without organomegaly. Extremities: no cyanosis. Neurologic: alert, active but irritable, with no motor or sensory deficits.

Laboratory Findings: WBC 8,400/μl, Hct 42.6%. Pulse oximetry (room air): 94%. Chest radiograph: see below.

Questions: What is the most likely diagnosis in this patient? What direct and supportive therapy should be given?

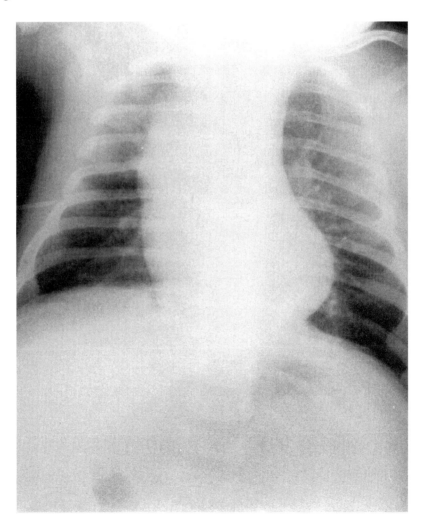

Diagnosis: Bronchiolitis with respiratory syncytial virus.

Discussion: Acute bronchiolitis is a form of viral respiratory tract infection and is seen most often in infants under 1 year old. Very young infants and those with underlying cardiorespiratory disorders are at particular risk of respiratory failure and death. The respiratory syncytial virus (RSV) is the most common cause of the syndrome.

RSV is the major respiratory pathogen of young children and is the major cause of lower respiratory disease in infants. RSV is transmitted primarily by close contact with contaminated fingers or fomites and by self-inoculation of the conjunctiva or anterior nares. Virus is also spread by coarse aerosols produced by coughing or sneezing. The incubation period of illness is approximately 4–6 days and virus shedding can last for 2 weeks or longer in children.

RSV infection leads to a wide spectrum of respiratory illnesses. In infants, 25–40% of infections result in lower respiratory tract involvement, including pneumonia, bronchiolitis, and tracheobronchitis. Many patients with RSV infection have **pneumonia**; however, the classic clinical syndrome is **bronchiolitis**. The illness typically begins with rhinorrhea and a low-grade fever progressing to a harsh cough and wheezing. Most patients gradually recover in 1–2 weeks. In more severe illness, tachypnea and dyspnea develop with inspiratory and/or expiratory retractions. The patient has difficulty feeding and can become markedly irritable or even lethargic. **Hypoxemia** is a frequent complication of RSV infection and patients should be assessed with pulse oximetry and monitored if they are hypoxemic.

Physical examination reveals an increased respiratory rate, prolonged expiration with retractions, and abdominal breathing. A rounded or barrel-shaped chest may be evident. Diffuse wheezing may be heard upon auscultation, but on occasion there may be no air movement because of severe obstruction. Cyanosis signals overt respiratory failure. The chest x-ray shows hyperexpansion, peribronchial thickening, and variable infiltrates ranging from diffuse interstitial to lobar or segmental consolidation.

The diagnosis of RSV infection is suspected on the basis of the epidemiologic setting, such as a severe illness in infants during an outbreak of RSV in the community. The specific diagnosis is established by isolation of RSV from respiratory secretions, including sputum, throat swabs, or nasopharyngeal washes. Virus is detected in tissue culture and identified by immunologic reactions employing immunofluorescence, enzyme-linked immunosorbent assay (ELISA), or other techniques.

Treatment for lower respiratory tract infections consists of respiratory therapy including hydration, suctioning of secretions, humidified oxygen, and beta-adrenergic pharmacologic agents as needed, for reversible airway obstruction. When severe hypoxemia is present, intubation and mechanical ventilatory support may be indicated.

Ribavirin, a synthetic nucleoside with broad-spectrum antiviral activity, is used for the treatment of lower respiratory tract disease due to RSV in the pediatric population. It has demonstrated a beneficial effect on the resolution of the disease, including an improvement in clinical scores, oxygenation, and a reduction in viral shedding. Aerosolized ribavirin appears to disrupt viral protein synthesis through inhibition of messenger RNA expression. Ribavirin is recommended for continuous aerosol administration with an oxygen hood or croupette, and more recently, with a ventilator using specific precautions, for 12–20 hours a day. It must be aerosolized using a specially designed aerosol generator known as a small particle aerosol generator (SPAG-2).

The present patient was treated with three doses of ribavirin using a SPAG-2 nebulizer in a 35% oxyhood for 3 days when the throat culture revealed RSV. His condition stabilized, becoming afebrile without tachypnea or other breathing difficulties. His appetite returned and he was discharged 6 days following admission.

Clinical Pearls

1. Approximately 0.5–2% of infants with severe lower respiratory tract disease require hospitalization and medical intervention, and most of these infants are less than 6 months of age.

2. The administration of aerosolized ribavirin to the mechanically ventilated infant mandates the use of special precautions to prevent complications and reduce the risk of crystalline precipitation in the circuit and subsequent ventilator dysfunction.

3. More than 50% of infants are infected with RSV during their first year of life, and close to 100% are infected during their first three years.

REFERENCES

1. King JC Jr, Burke AR, Clemens JD, et al. Respiratory syncytial virus illnesses in HIV-infected and noninfected children. Pediatr Infect Dis J 1993;12:733–739.
2. Chipps BE, Sullivan WF, Portnoy JM. Alpha-2A-interferon for treatment of bronchiolitis caused by respiratory syncytial virus. Pediatr Infect Dis J 1993;12:653–658.
3. American Academy of Pediatrics, Committee on Infectious Diseases: Use of ribavirin in the treatment of respiratory syncytial virus infection. Pediatrics 1993;92:501–504.
4. Kacmarek RM, Kratohvil J. Evaluation of a double-enclosure double-vacuum unit scavenging system for ribavirin administration. Respir Care 1992;37:37–45.
5. Stretton M, Ajizian SJ, Mitchell I, et al. Intensive care course and outcome of patients infected with respiratory syncytial virus. Pediatr Pulmonol 1992;13:143–150.
6. Smith DW, Frankel LR, Mathers LH, et al. A controlled trial of aerosolized ribavirin in infants receiving mechanical ventilation for severe respiratory syncytial virus infection. New Engl J Med 1991;325:24–29.

PATIENT 38

A 73-year-old woman with epistaxis and blurred vision

A 73-year-old woman presented for evaluation with a complaint of epistaxis which had occurred sporadically over a one-month period. In the past week she had developed blurred vision as well. Her past medical history included hypertension, congestive heart failure, coronary artery disease, hypothyroidism, diverticulitis, and a 75-pack-year cigarette smoking history. Her medications included isosorbide, levothyroxine, captopril, furosemide, digoxin, potassium chloride, alprazolam, and nortriptyline.

Physical Examination: Temperature 98.9°; pulse 80; respirations 16; blood pressure 126/76. HEENT: pink mucosa without polyps or deviated septum. Chest: clear. Cardiac: regular rhythm without murmurs. Abdomen: soft, without masses or organomegaly. Extremities: no clubbing or cyanosis. Neurologic: nonfocal.

Laboratory Findings: WBC 8,790/μl, Hct 29.6%, platelets 354,000/μl. PT 12.6 sec (control 11.9 sec), PTT 19.9 sec. ABG (room air): pH 7.37, pCO_2 46 mmHg, pO_2 66 mmHg, SaO_2 95%. Chest radiograph: see below.

Question: What is the likely cause of epistaxis in this patient?

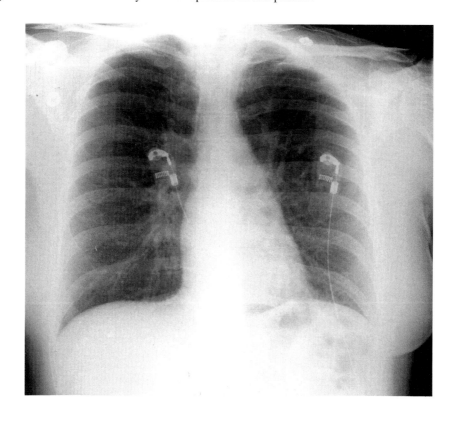

Answer: Nasopharyngeal carcinoma.

Discussion: Carcinomas of the head and neck account for 40,000 new cases of cancer each year in the United States, and because of their propensity to cause symptoms early in the course of their development, they are often curable tumors. Risk factors for development of cancer of the head and neck are identical to those for other tumors of the aerodigestive tract, with alcohol consumption and tobacco use being the most important. Smokeless (or chewing) tobacco has also been associated with the development of head and neck carcinoma.

The overwhelming majority of cancers of the head and neck, including nasopharyngeal carcinoma, are **squamous cell tumors**. The nasopharynx, the anatomic region located between the soft palate and the tongue, is lined with pseudostratified, ciliated, columnar epithelium and serves to filter and humidify dry inspired gases. Nasopharyngeal carcinoma originates from epithelial cells of the nasopharynx and frequently arises in the fossa of Rosenmüller. Interestingly, unlike other head and neck cancers, nasopharyngeal cancers do not seem to be related to the use of tobacco and alcohol. Rather, nasopharyngeal cancer has an interesting association with **Epstein-Barr virus** (EBV) infection, and evidence of EBV can be found in the malignant tissue of 90% of nasopharyngeal cancers.

The three histologic types of nasopharyngeal carcinomas that have been accepted by the World Health Organization (WHO) include: squamous cell carcinoma (WHO type 1), nonkeratinizing carcinoma (WHO type 2), and undifferentiated carcinoma (WHO type 3). The WHO type 3 tumor is the most common, and though it is sometimes called a lymphoepithelioma, it arises from squamous epithelium. Because the nasopharynx, including its epithelium, lymphoid tissue, and supporting structures, contains a wide variety of cell types, many different lesions may occur.

A primary tumor of the nasopharynx may obstruct the posterior choana, resulting in blood-tinged nasal drainage. Cranial neuropathies are reported in 20% of patients with nasopharyngeal carcinoma and result from superior extension of the tumor and the petrosphenoidal crossway formed by the foramen lacerum from the fossa of Rosenmüller into the cranium. Despite the fact that many nasopharyngeal carcinomas are diagnosed early, distant metastases will develop in 25% of cases, and the lungs, bones, and liver are favored sites for spread of the primary tumor. As patients with head and neck cancers are at a very high risk for developing primary bronchogenic carcinoma (at the rate of up to 4% per year), a new lung lesion in a patient with otherwise controlled disease should be carefully evaluated for a potentially curable lung lesion.

The mainstay of treatment for patients with nasopharyngeal carcinoma is high-dose **radiation therapy**, and the likelihood of cure with this modality is directly related to the size of the primary tumor and spread to regional lymph nodes. Small tumors have an 80–90% cure rate with radiation therapy, and the role of surgery has been limited. The presence of cranial nerve involvement classifies the primary tumor as a T4 lesion, making the disease a stage IV cancer. The ultimate prognosis for this stage is poor, and therapy consists of high-dose or superfractionated radiotherapy of the primary tumor and clinically involved regional lymph nodes. Neoadjuvant chemotherapy (chemotherapy given at the time of radiation) is also employed by some physicians.

The present patient underwent radiation and chemotherapy and is presently an outpatient receiving follow-up cancer care at an oncology clinic.

Clinical Pearls

1. Carcinoma of the nasopharynx is infrequent in the United States, where it comprises 4% of head and neck malignancies.

2. Unlike other head and neck cancers, nasopharyngeal carcinoma is not related to tobacco and alcohol use. Epstein-Barr virus is an important factor in the development of this tumor.

3. The primary treatment for all nasopharyngeal carcinomas, regardless of stage, is radiation therapy.

REFERENCES

1. Fandi A, Altun M, Azli N, et al. Nasopharyngeal cancer: Epidemiology, staging, and treatment. Semin Oncol 1994;21:382–397.
2. Feinmesser R, Miyazaki I, Cheung R, et al. Diagnosis of nasopharyngeal carcinoma by DNA amplification of tissue obtained by fine-needle aspiration. N Engl J Med 1992;326:17–21.
3. Bailet JW, Mark RJ, Abemayor E, et al. Nasopharyngeal carcinoma: Treatment results with primary radiation therapy. Laryngoscope 1992;102:965–972.

PATIENT 39

A 32-year-old man with increasing shortness of breath for 18 months

A 32-year-old man with an 18-month history of episodic shortness of breath presented to his physician complaining of increased shortness of breath for 7 days. Past medical history included gastroesophageal reflux disease and asthma. Medications included cisapride, omeprazole, and albuterol. He had been a cave explorer in West Virginia until 3 years ago.

Physical Examination: Temperature 99.6°; pulse 95; respirations 24; blood pressure 110/70. Chest: clear to auscultation. Cardiac: regular rhythm without murmurs. Abdomen: without masses or organomegaly. Extremities: no clubbing or cyanosis. Neurologic: nonfocal.

Laboratory Findings: ABG (room air): pH 7.40; pCO_2 39 mmHg, pO_2 66 mmHg, HCO_3^- 24 mEq/L, SaO_2 91%. Chest radiograph: see below left. Chest CT (see below right): severe tracheal narrowing. PFTs: FVC .47 L (10% predicted), FEV_1 .18 L (5% predicted), FEF_{25-75} 0.14 L/sec (3% predicted), FRC 1.60 L (33% predicted).

Question: What is the cause of this patient's dyspnea?

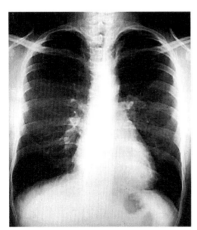 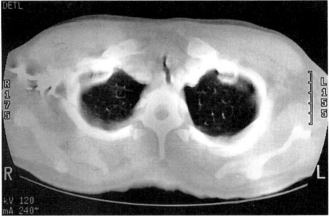

Diagnosis: Mediastinal fibrosis and upper airway obstruction secondary to histoplasmosis.

Discussion: Histoplasma capsulatum is a dimorphic fungus that grows as a **mold** at room temperature. Hyphae bear both large and small spores that can be used for identification; despite its name, the fungus is unencapsulated. Infection has been encountered in many areas of the world, although within the United States infection is most common in the southeastern, mid-Atlantic, and central states. Endemic areas are probably determined by the availability of proper conditions in nature for the growth of the fungus. *H. capsulatum* prefers moist surface soil, particularly when it is enriched by nitrogen-containing droppings of certain birds and bats. The fungus also has been isolated after exposure to dust by raking, bulldozing, cleaning dirt-floored chicken coops, or cave exploring. It has been estimated that 50 million people in the south-central United States have been infected with the fungus, with 500,000 new cases occurring annually.

The pathogenesis of histoplasmosis is as follows: **spores** are inhaled into the lungs, and some reach the alveolar spaces, where they are converted to the yeast phase of the organism. The yeast forms then multiply and grow within macrophages and disseminate via the bloodstream. Eventually, a T-lymphocyte response is mounted, granuloma formation occurs, and the infection is controlled. Granulomas can develop fibrosis, and **calcification** in the lungs, liver, and spleen is common.

Clinical syndromes of histoplasmosis range from the completely asymptomatic to brief, self-limited episodes resembling influenza to miliary-type illnesses (primarily in persons with significant immunocompromise, such as AIDS patients). In the self-limited form of the disease (the most common manifestation), chest radiographs usually show a focal infiltrate with significant ipsilateral hilar adenopathy. The infiltrate may eventually scar down, calcify, and resemble a pulmonary nodule that can be mistaken for a carcinoma.

Diagnosis of histoplasmosis is often not made, as the disease is **self-limited** and many patients do not seek medical attention. It is difficult to demonstrate the organisms directly from respiratory secretions, and the histoplasmin antigen skin test cannot distinguish acute disease from past infection. A variety of serologic tests is available, though the sensitivity and specificity is not ideal. In immunocompetent hosts, recovery without therapy is the rule. In AIDS patients with disseminated disease, antifungal therapy with amphotericin B or one of the oral imidazoles is indicated.

A feared complication of histoplasmosis is **fibrosing mediastinitis**, in which some or all of the mediastinal structures, including the trachea, major bronchi, superior vena cava, pulmonary veins, and pulmonary arteries may become encased in dense fibrous tissue. A variety of clinical syndromes may result, including the superior vena cava syndrome, cor pulmonale and pulmonary hypertension, and fixed upper airway obstruction. When symptoms are caused by a few lymph nodes that have undergone fibrosis and then compressed adjacent structures, occasionally there is regression and improvement. However, when there is diffuse mediastinal fibrosis, few therapeutic options exist. Drug treatment is not successful, as the fibrosis is an immunologically mediated response, rather than the result of active infection. Surgery is extremely difficult in these cases and not likely to be associated with a good outcome.

The pulmonary function tests of the present patient demonstrated severe airflow obstruction, and the CT scan showed severe narrowing of the trachea. Combined with his history of cave exploring and splenic and hepatic calcifications seen on CT scan (cuts not shown), a diagnosis of mediastinal fibrosis secondary to histoplasmosis was made.

Clinical Pearls

1. *H. capsulatum*, one of the so-called geographic fungi, is found in the south-central United States as well as in western Pennsylvania, Ohio, and West Virginia.

2. Most infections with *H. capsulatum* that occur in immunocompetent hosts are self-limited and relatively benign infections resembling viral syndromes and upper respiratory illnesses.

3. Progressive disseminated histoplasmosis, seen now most commonly in AIDS patients, is a life-threatening disorder that requires specific antifungal therapy.

4. Mediastinal fibrosis is an uncommon but potentially life-threatening form of the disease, with no specific therapy.

REFERENCES

1. Sherrick AD, Brown LR, Harms GF, Myers JL. The radiographic findings of fibrosing mediastinitis. Chest 1994;106:484–489.
2. Wheat J. Histoplasmosis: Recognition and treatment. Clin Infect Dis 1994;Suppl 1:S19–27.
3. Sharkey-Mathis PK, Velez J, Fetchick R, Graybill JR. Histoplasmosis in the acquired immunodeficiency syndrome (AIDS): Treatment with itraconazole and fluconazole. J Acquir Immune Defic Syndr 1993;6:809–819.
4. Wheat LJ, Connolly-Stringfield P, Williams B, et al. Diagnosis of histoplasmosis in patients with the acquired immunodeficiency syndrome by detection of *Histoplasma capsulatum* polysaccharide antigen in bronchoalveolar lavage fluid. Am Rev Respir Dis 1992;145:1421–1424.
5. Loyd JE, Tillman BF, Atkinson JB, et al. Mediastinal fibrosis complicating histoplasmosis. Medicine 1988;67:295–310.

PATIENT 40

A 17-year-old developmentally delayed girl with difficulty breathing

A 17-year-old developmentally delayed girl presented to the pediatric clinic with difficulty breathing. Past medical history included pyloric stenosis, nemaline myopathy, and severe scoliosis. Seven years ago she suffered respiratory arrest and has required nocturnal ventilatory support since.

Physical Examination: Temperature 98.6°; pulse 96; respirations 28; blood pressure 118/62. Chest: air entry fair, without wheezes or rales, Size 6 fenestrated tracheostomy tube in place. Cardiac: regular rhythm, without murmurs. Abdomen: without masses or organomegaly. Extremities: no cyanosis or clubbing. Neurologic: severe weakness, all muscle groups, with patient confined to a wheelchair.

Laboratory Findings: ABG (room air): pH 7.33, pCO_2 46 mmHg, pO_2 75 mmHg, HCO_3^- 22 mEq/L, SaO_2 96%. PFTs: V_t 180 ml, f = 22, VC 600 ml, NIF –18 cm H_2O. Chest radiograph: severe scoliosis with flattened bilateral hemidiaphragms.

Question: What are the respiratory considerations in the care of the patient with nemaline myopathy?

Discussion: Neuromuscular diseases, whether fixed or progressive, acute or chronic, are often associated with respiratory insufficiency, usually resulting from diaphragmatic weakness or fatigue. In addition, a great deal of the morbidity and mortality associated with neuromuscular disease can be attributed to respiratory complications, including hypercapnic respiratory failure, pulmonary embolism arising from venous thrombosis caused by immobilization, and most significantly **pneumonia**. Pneumonias can develop in neuromuscular disease patients through several mechanisms. Weakness of the respiratory muscles and diaphragms can lead to ineffective cough and inability to clear secretions, allowing colonization of the lower respiratory tract with potential pathogens, including enteric gram-negative rods. In addition, if bulbar muscles are involved, patients are prone to aspiration and pneumonia.

Nemaline myopathy is a rare congenital disorder distinguished from the muscular dystrophies by the presence of rods or coils of thread-like structures in muscle fibers. Some infants with the disease demonstrate severe respiratory weakness and hypotonia, and early death from respiratory complications may ensue. More commonly, however, children with this disease have a relatively benign, non-progressive course with weakness, hypotonia, and delayed motor development. A narrow face, high-arched palate, kyphoscoliosis, and club feet are characteristic. The weakness tends to be more severe proximally, but may be less severe than suggested by the reduced muscle bulk. The extraocular muscles tend to be spared despite involvement of the facial, palatal, and pharyngeal muscles.

Although it is rare for the disease to be first recognized in adult life, there is a wide spectrum of severity, and some adult patients are asymptomatic. Others have had mild weakness since childhood, and still others manifest progressive weakness. Some adults have severe wasting of distal leg muscles and fatal cardiomyopathy sometimes is seen. The disease may be fatal in infancy or childhood as well. In some cases, **nocturnal hypoventilation** may be present. It is attributed to a defect in the medulla and nocturnal ventilatory support may be used to treat the central sleep apnea. Therefore, most patients with nemaline myopathy who present with respiratory failure require temporary ventilatory support.

There are several **ventilatory support** options in patients with neuromuscular disease. If total lung and chest wall compliance are normal, the patient potentially can be managed with negative-pressure noninvasive ventilation, such as a poncho wrap or chest cuirass. However, if secretions are a major problem or if chest wall compliance is not normal, the pressures generated by a negative-pressure ventilator may not be adequate, and positive pressure may be required. This can initially be achieved with noninvasive strategies, such as CPAP or BiPAP, but if the respiratory failure is severe or prolonged, permanent ventilatory support may be needed. Such permanent support is usually best provided through a tracheostomy.

The present patient underwent a nighttime sleep study that demonstrated significant desaturations. She was placed on nighttime ventilatory support with CPAP, and her desaturations resolved. In addition, she noted much less shortness of breath during the day.

Clinical Pearls

1. Diagnosis of nemaline myopathy is based on demonstration of the characteristic nemaline rods in skeletal muscles.

2. Although nemaline myopathy affects all muscles, including the diaphragm, it is typically not responsible for fatal ventilatory failure.

3. Severe nocturnal respiratory failure, caused by a defect in the central control of breathing, is a characteristic of nemaline myopathy.

REFERENCES
1. Falga-Tirado C, Perez-Peman P, Ordi-Ros J, Bofill JM, Balcells E. Adult onset of nemaline myopathy presenting as respiratory insufficiency, Respiration 1995;62:353–354.
2. Bergmann M, Kamarampaka M, Kuchelmeister K, Klein H, Koch H. Nemaline myopathy: Two autopsy reports. Childs Nerv Syst 1995;11:610–615.
3. Wallgen-Pettersson C, Rapola J, Donner M. Pathology of congenital nemaline myopathy: A follow-up study. J Neurol Sci 1988;83:243–257.
4. Maayan CH, Springer C, Armon Y, et al. Nemaline myopathy as a cause of sleep hypoventilation. Pediatrics 1986;77:390–395.

PATIENT 41

A 38-year-old man with exertional dyspnea and lower extremity edema

A 38-year-old morbidly obese man presented to his physician's office complaining of unusual exertional dyspnea with lower extremity edema. His symptoms had been progressive over the previous 2 months. Past medical history included obstructive sleep apnea, a 38-pack-year smoking history, and bipolar psychiatric disorder.

Physical Examination: Temperature 98.6°; pulse 88; respirations 20; blood pressure 150/95. Chest: clear to auscultation. Cardiac: jugular venous distension present, regular rate and rhythm with accentuated S2 at the right sternal border. Abdomen: without masses or organomegaly. Extremities: ++ pitting edema of ankles bilaterally, without clubbing or cyanosis.

Laboratory Findings: ABG (room air): pH 7.39, pCO_2 50 mmHg, pO_2 67 mmHg, HCO_3^- 29 mEq/L, SaO_2 93%. EKG: right axis deviation, right atrial enlargement, and right ventricular hypertrophy. PFTs: FVC 3.65 L (73% predicted), FEV_1 3.55 (92% predicted), PEFR 6.81 L/sec (75% predicted), RV 1.87 L (96% predicted), TLC 5.73 L (85% predicted). Chest radiograph (see below): cardiomegaly with prominent pulmonary arteries.

Question: What is the likely cause of this patient's dyspnea and leg swelling?

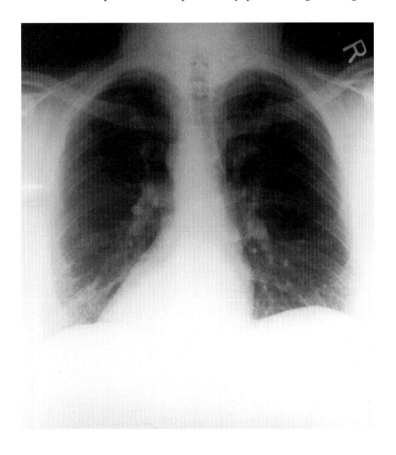

Answer: Obesity-hypoventilation syndrome.

Discussion: Sleep disordered breathing is increasingly recognized as a common condition affecting many patients. Several primary disorders have been described, and it also is well known that abnormal breathing during sleep can complicate a variety of other medical conditions, such as congestive heart failure and stroke.

Syndromes of sleep disordered breathing include central sleep apnea, obstructive sleep apnea, the upper airway resistance syndrome, and the obesity-hypoventilation syndrome, also sometimes referred to as the "Pickwickian syndrome," after the character Joe in Dickens' novel *The Pickwick Papers*. The **upper airway resistance syndrome** is characterized by loud snoring and increased resistance to airflow in the upper airway, though apneas and desaturations are not seen. **Central sleep apnea** is defined as apnea occurring without any respiratory efforts at all, as evidenced by a lack of contraction of the respiratory muscles at a time when airflow at the nose is absent. This type of apnea is uncommon. The **obstructive sleep apnea syndrome** (OSAS) is manifest by lack of airflow and oxygen desaturations occurring while respiratory efforts are being made.

Patients with OSAS are usually obese, and the pathogenesis of the syndrome is felt to be related to a loss of neuromuscular tone in the upper airway that occurs mainly during REM sleep. Because of the repeated apneas, patients are awakened throughout the night and have fragmented and interrupted sleep, leading to the characteristic complaint of daytime hypersomnolence. In true OSAS, apneas and desaturations occur only during sleep; during wakefulness there is no evidence of hypoxemia or hypercarbia.

Systemic hypertension commonly accompanies OSAS, but daytime hypoxia leading to pulmonary hypertension and cor pulmonale is unusual, *except* in patients with the obesity-hypoventilation syndrome. Though there is some overlap between patients with obesity-hypoventilation and OSAS, not all patients with obesity-hypoventilation have nighttime obstructive events, indicating that there likely is a difference in the underlying pathology of the two syndromes. The development of hypercarbia in obesity-hypoventilation patients probably is related to a combination of mechanical impedance to breathing and a defect in the central ventilatory drive.

Obesity may also have effects on pulmonary function independent of co-morbid conditions such as OSAS or hypoventilation. Usually, pulmonary function abnormalities are mild, with the most consistent finding a reduction in the expiratory reserve volume, and a smaller reduction in functional residual capacity. Gas exchange should be normal unless airway obstruction is present. Ventilatory drive abnormalities have been noted in simple obesity, with the CO_2 response 60% of normal on average and the resting respiratory rate 40% above normal. A mild degree of arterial hypoxemia is present in many obese patients, and this finding tends to be worse when the patient is supine, perhaps due to the abdomen compressing the diaphragm and causing atelectasis and increased ventilation/perfusion mismatching.

The present patient was suspected on clinical grounds of having Pickwickian (obesity-hypoventilation) syndrome, and he demonstrated a blunted respiratory drive during a CO_2 provocation test. In addition, nighttime polysomnography revealed episodes consistent with obstructive sleep apnea. Application of positive airway pressure improved his apneic episodes, and he is currently maintained on BiPAP therapy at night.

Clinical Pearls

1. Disordered breathing is a feature of several important clinical syndromes, including central sleep apnea, obstructive sleep apnea, and the obesity-hypoventilation syndrome.

2. Patients with pure obstructive sleep apnea are usually eucapnic during the day, whereas those with obesity-hypoventilation can manifest hypoxia, hypercarbia, and eventually pulmonary hypertension with cor pulmonale.

3. Obesity can lead to (usually mild) abnormalities in pulmonary function and gas exchange, even in the absence of concomitant hypoventilation.

REFERENCES

1. Strohl KP, Redline S. Recognition of obstructive sleep apnea. Am J Respir Crit Care Med 1996;154:279–289.
2. Strollo PJ Jr, Rogers RM. Obstructive sleep apnea. New Engl J Med 1996;334:99–104.
3. Martin TJ, Sanders MH. Chronic alveolar hypoventilation: A review for the clinician. Sleep 1995;18:617–634.
4. Grunstein RR, Wilcox I. Sleep-disordered breathing and obesity. Baillieres Clin Endocrinol Metab 1994;8:601–628.
5. Young T, Palta M, Dempsey J, et al. The occurrence of sleep-disordered breathing among middle-aged adults. New Engl J Med 1993;328:1230–1235.
6. Kopelman PG. Sleep apnea and hypoventilation in obesity. Int J Obes Relat Metab Disord 1992;16 suppl 2:S37–42.

PATIENT 42

A 1-year-old boy with cough and vomiting following a brief period of submersion

A 1-year-old boy was brought to the emergency department by his mother after being submersed in water in the bathtub for approximately 1 minute. He was being supervised by his 9-year-old sister when he was found unresponsive and not breathing. The boy had been previously well.

Physical Examination: Temperature 97°; pulse 130; respirations 28; blood pressure 90/50. HEENT: clear nasal discharge. Chest: scattered rhonchi bilaterally. Cardiac: tachycardic. Abdomen: bowel sounds present. Neurologic: alert and crying.

Laboratory Findings: WBC 16,500/μl, Hct 35%. PT 14.5 sec, PTT 35.0 sec, control 11.1 sec. Na^+ 133 mEq/L, K^+ 3.0 mEq/L, Cl^- 101 mEq/L, HCO_2 8 mEq/L. Glucose 257 mg/dl, BUN 4 mg/dl. ABG (room air): pH 7.13, pCO_2 31 mmHg, pO_2 122 mmHg, HCO_3^- 10 mEq/L, SaO_2 97%. Chest radiograph: see below.

Questions: What is the cause of the acidosis in this patient? What are the general and respiratory care considerations in the management of this patient?

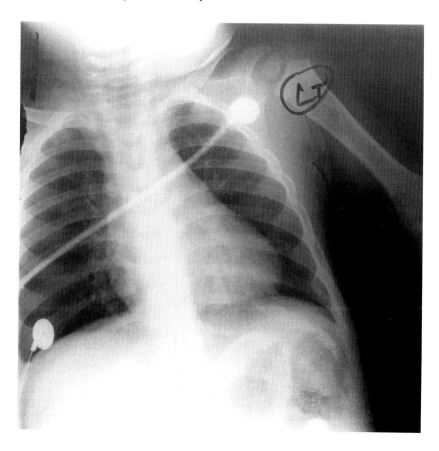

Diagnosis: Near-drowning.

Discussion: Near-drowning, with or without aspiration, is to suffocate by submersion in water and to survive for at least 24 hours. (The term "drowning" is reserved for those unfortunate persons who die as a result of submersion.) Approximately 7,000 individuals drown in the United States each year, and that is only a small proportion of the total number of near-drowning events. Drowning is an important cause of death in children, with many accidents occurring in backyard swimming pools.

The morbidity and mortality associated with drowning and near-drowning are related to the sequence of events that occur with submersion. **Laryngospasm** occurs initially, and although asphyxia can result if the spasm does not remit, the usual course is that the victim eventually takes an involuntary breath and **aspirates water** into the lungs. This can cause pulmonary edema, shunting, ventilation/perfusion imbalance, and acute respiratory distress syndrome (ARDS). In addition, systemic hypoxia that develops can lead to anoxic encephalopathy and systemic tissue acidosis.

Original theories suggested that aspiration of hypotonic fresh water resulted in the transudation of fluid from the lungs into the intravascular space, causing severe fluid overload with dilution of serum electrolytes. Also, it was suggested that hypertonic salt water resulted in the osmotic shifting of water from the intravascular space into the lungs, causing pulmonary edema and hypertonic serum. It now is clear that fresh water aspiration changes the surface tension properties of lung surfactant, leading to alveolar instability and atelectasis. This results in ventilation/perfusion mismatching with perfusion of unventilated lung segments (intrapulmonary shunt). Salt water aspiration leads to persistent fluid-filled alveoli that cause perfusion of unventilated lung segments.

Although these electrolyte and volume abnormalities have been shown, their existence is dependent on the amount of fluid aspirated. As most drowning victims aspirate only a small amount of fluid, these volume shifts usually are not clinically significant, and there are few management issues that hinge on the type of water in which the patient was submerged. Regardless of mechanism, all fresh and salt water drownings result in arterial **hypoxemia** secondary to **ventilation/perfusion mismatching** and **intrapulmonary shunting**.

The treatment of all drowning and near-drowning victims includes stabilizing respiratory and cardiac functions, making timely neurologic assessments, and observing for secondary signs and symptoms of pneumonia. CPR should be instituted immediately at the scene. *All* victims, regardless of how well they appear, should be admitted for at least 24 hours of observation because post-submersion sequelae, including the development of ARDS, often have late onset manifestations. Oxygen should be administered as a matter of routine until adequacy of arterial oxygenation can be assessed.

The present patient was removed from the water within 1 minute of submersion. Upon detection of breathlessness, CPR was given by the patient's mother. The boy responded by beginning to cry and was admitted to the hospital for overnight observation. His laboratory findings were consistent with a lactic acidosis which occurred as a result of tissue hypoxia, and they resolved quickly once oxygen was administered and the boy's respiratory status stabilized. He was discharged the following day without post-incident sequelae.

Clinical Pearls

1. In the United States, drowning is the second leading cause of injury in children older than 9 months of age.

2. Approximately 10–15% of drowning victims experience persistent laryngospasm, while 85–90% experience laryngeal relaxation with aspiration of water and gastric contents.

3. Regardless of mechanism, all fresh and salt water drownings result in arterial hypoxemia secondary to ventilation/perfusion mismatching and intrapulmonary shunting, and severe hypoxia is the major cause of morbidity and mortality related to submersion.

REFERENCES
1. Noonan L, Howrey R, Ginsburg CM. Freshwater submersion injuries in children: A retrospective review of seventy-five hospitalized patients. Pediatrics 1996;98:368–371.
2. Kallas HJ, O'Rourke PP. Drowning and immersion injuries in children. Curr Opin Pediatr 1993;5:295–302.
3. Modell JH. Drowning. New Engl J Med 1993;328:253–256.
4. Quan L. Drowning issues in resuscitation. Ann Emerg Med 1993;22:366–369.
5. Fields AI. Near-drowning in the pediatric population. Crit Care Clin 1992;8:113–129.

PATIENT 43

A 9-year-old girl with progressive dyspnea

A 9-year-old girl presented in her physician's office with shortness of breath. At 2 months of age, she developed respiratory failure due to overwhelming viral pneumonia, and she required a prolonged hospital stay. As a consequence of her initial infection, respiratory distress, and mechanical ventilation, she developed pulmonary fibrosis. Her medications at present included prednisone, cyclophosphamide, iron, and multivitamins.

Physical Examination: Temperature 98.6°; pulse 105; respirations 30, using accessory muscles; blood pressure 120/63. Chest: bilateral coarse crackles with expiratory wheezes over the base of the lung. Tracheostomy in place. Cardiac: tachycardic, without murmurs. Abdomen: without masses or organomegaly. Extremities: no cyanosis. Neurologic: alert and oriented, nonfocal.

Laboratory Findings: ABG (28% ventimask): pH 7.35, pCO_2 42 mmHg, pO_2 64 mmHg, HCO_3^- 22 mEq/L, SaO_2 89%. Chest radiograph: bilateral, diffuse reticulonodular densities.

Course: In the physician's office, the patient was treated with aerosolized albuterol. The mother refused the physician's recommendation of hospitalization for further medical evaluation.

Question: To what can this patient's lung disease be attributed?

Diagnosis: Pulmonary fibrosis due to oxygen toxicity.

Discussion: Interstitial fibrosis is a process in which the normal interstitium is damaged and replaced by an increased number of mesenchymal cells and their connective tissue products. This fibrosis results from chronic inflammatory disorders of the lung parenchyma. Irreversible destruction of normal lung architecture is an expected outcome. The accumulation of immune and inflammatory effector cells within the interstitium and alveolar air spaces seems to be the precursor of both parenchymal injury and subsequent fibrosis.

The two histologic patterns associated with interstitial pulmonary fibrosis are **desquamative interstitial pneumonitis** (DIP) and **usual interstitial pneumonitis** (UIP). The two patterns are not mutually exclusive and features of each may be found in the same biopsy specimens. The relationship between UIP and DIP is not clearly defined, although two distinct variants of the disease are evident. Some authorities view the two entities as sequential components of the same disease process, with DIP representing the earlier, more inflammatory phase.

The fibrotic process in the lungs produces characteristic abnormalities in pulmonary performance, and interstitial fibrosis is the prototypical restrictive lung disease, with characteristic **low lung volumes** (particularly total lung capacity, vital capacity, and functional residual capacity) and diffusing capacity seen on pulmonary function testing. In addition, invasion of the interstitial spaces and alveoli by inflammatory cells and fibroblasts eventually compromises lung compliance. The lung volumes decrease and the work of breathing increases. In response, the pattern of breathing in patients with idiopathic pulmonary fibrosis is rapid and shallow. **Hyperventilation**, a characteristic response to noncompliant lungs, maintains the alveolar and arterial pCO_2 at low levels through most of the course of fibrosis. In the advanced stages of the disease, as ventilation-perfusion mismatching becomes extreme, **hypercapnia** prevails.

Airflow obstruction is *not* a feature of idiopathic pulmonary fibrosis. Indeed, expiratory flow rates at a particular lung volume are increased (patients may have a supernormal FEV_1/FVC ratio) because of the increased elastic recoil of the lungs. The finding of an obstructive defect suggests an additional diagnosis.

Arterial hypoxemia occurs at first only during exertion and later while at rest. Hypoxemia at rest is due predominantly to ventilation-perfusion mismatch. During exercise, impaired diffusion contributes to worsening hypoxemia; the transit time of blood through the capillary network quickens, leaving insufficient time for diffusion of oxygen through the thickened alveolar-capillary membrane.

In many cases of pulmonary fibrosis, no underlying cause is found, and the disease process is termed idiopathic. However, in the present case the patient's history of prolonged mechanical ventilation suggests oxygen toxicity as a major contributor to the development of fibrosis. The toxicity of **high inspired oxygen tensions** has been recognized for a long time. Acutely, breathing 100% oxygen can cause tracheobronchitis, which generally subsides without lasting injury. Over a longer period of exposure, it has been shown that breathing inspired oxygen tensions of > 0.5 atmospheres (atm) is associated with an increased risk of O_2 toxicity, manifest as diffuse alveolar damage and pulmonary fibrosis. Such significant toxicity becomes more common with higher inspired O_2 tensions, and may be seen commonly after breathing 0.8–1.0 atm of oxygen for 1–2 weeks. Though the exact mechanism of oxygen-induced lung disease is unknown, many investigators feel that the generation of toxic species such as superoxide radical and hydrogen peroxide is the important inciting event.

The best defense against pulmonary oxygen toxicity is to avoid high inspired O_2 tensions by correcting the underlying disorder as quickly as possible and by judicious use of PEEP. Locally administered antioxidants and exogenous surfactant have not been shown to be of benefit. Immunosuppressive therapy with corticosteroids or agents such as cyclophosphamide may benefit some patients with idiopathic fibrosis.

The present patient, having declined further evaluation, left the office without additional follow up.

Clinical Pearls

1. Prolonged administration of oxygen at high concentrations is associated with a risk of lung disease, including interstitial edema, hyaline membrane formation, and proliferation of type II alveolar pneumocytes.

2. Oxygen concentration of > 0.5 atmospheres has been associated with toxicity, though the risk of lung damage rises with higher concentrations used for prolonged periods.

3. Oxygen toxicity is felt to occur because of the generation of free radicals and other toxic oxygen species, though administration of antioxidants to patients at risk does not seem to prevent or ameliorate the development of this condition. Use of PEEP, low inspired O_2 tensions, and correction of the underlying pulmonary disorder are the best approaches to avoid this complication.

REFERENCES

1. Pfenninger J. Acute respiratory distress syndrome (ARDS) in neonates and children. Pediatr Anaesth 1996;6:173–181.
2. Russell GA. Antioxidants and neonatal lung disease. Eur J Pediatr 1994;153: S36–41.
3. Fan LL. Evaluation and therapy of chronic interstitial pneumonitis in children. Curr Opin Pediatr 1994;6:248–254.
4. Bokulic RE, Hillman BC. Interstitial lung disease in children. Pediatr Clin North Am 1994;41:543–567.
5. Tsan MF. Superoxide dismutase and pulmonary oxygen toxicity. Proc Soc Exp Biol Med 1993;203:286–290.

PATIENT 44

A 44-year-old man with progressive fatigue and recent shortness of breath

A 44-year-old man was referred to a pulmonologist by his private physician for progressive fatigue and shortness of breath. As a firefighter, his occupational history included exposure to smoke, heat, toxic gases, and oxygen deficient environments for the previous 18 years.

Physical Examination: Temperature 98.6°; pulse 70; respirations 24; blood pressure 144/86. Chest: clear. Cardiac: regular rhythm without murmurs. Abdomen: without masses or organomegaly. Extremities: no clubbing or cyanosis. Neurologic: normal.

Laboratory Findings: ABG (room air): pH 7.39, pCO_2 39 mmHg, pO_2 88 mmHg, HCO_3^- 24 mEq/L. Exercise testing: the patient completed 8.25 minutes of incremental cycle ergometry stopping at a maximum workload of 200 watts due to lower extremity fatigue. PFTs: see below.

Question: How should this patient's pulmonary function tests be interpreted?

| | Pre Bronchodilator | | | Post Bronchodilator Challenge | | | |
| | | | | First Effort | | Second Effort | |
	Actual	Pred	% Pred	Actual	% Pred	Actual	% Pred
		Mechanics					
FVC	4.48 L	5.04 L	89%	4.44 L	88%	4.56 L	90%
FEV$_1$	3.76 L	3.97 L	95%	3.72 L	94%	3.80 L	96%
FEV$_1$/FVC	84%	78%	108%	84%	108%	83%	106%
PEF	9.92 L/S	9.56 L/S	104%	9.12 L/S	95%	8.96 L/S	94%
FEF$_{25-75\%}$	3.76 L/S	5.27 L/S	71%	3.60 L/S	68%	4.08 L/S	77%
		Volumes					
TLC	7.01 L	7.26 L	97%				
SVC	4.79 L	5.04 L	95%				
TGV	3.09 L	3.73 L	83%				
ERV	0.87 L	1.51 L	58%				
RV	2.22 L	2.22 L	100%				
RV/TLC	31%						
	Diffusing Capacity (Transfer Factor)						
DLCO	25.80	30.60	84%				

Diagnosis: Normal pulmonary function.

Discussion: Pulmonary function tests (PFTs) are among the most important and useful tools in the clinician's diagnostic bag for evaluating the complaint of dyspnea. Though the clinical history, physical examination, and radiographic studies are of great importance, PFTs can broadly classify the patient either as normal or as belonging to one (or more) of several disease categories and can provide objective, reproducible, and quantitative information regarding lung function.

Standard PFTs have three components: measurement of **lung volume**, measurement of **air flow**, and measurement of the **diffusing capacity** for carbon monoxide, used as a marker for oxygen diffusion. Results are compared to predicted values for normal, healthy, nonsmoking persons of body size similar to the patient's. Measured values should be 80% or greater of the predicted value. Lung volumes include total lung capacity, vital capacity, functional residual capacity, and residual volume. In the class of abnormalities known as the restrictive lung diseases (such as interstitial fibrosis, sarcoidosis, silicosis, and others), lung volumes are reduced. Diffusing capacity also tends to be reduced in these disorders, as the alveolar-capillary interface becomes thickened with inflammation and fibrosis. A drop in diffusing capacity is often the earliest physiologic manifestation of interstitial lung disease.

In the **obstructive lung diseases**, which are often characterized by hyperinflation and air trapping (such as emphysema or an acute asthma attack), lung volumes (particularly the total lung capacity and residual volume) are above predicted levels. In addition to hyperinflation seen with obstructive disease, patients with asthma, emphysema, and chronic bronchitis display the hallmark of airflow limitation: a reduced FEV_1/FVC ratio. Healthy individuals should be able to blow out 75% of a maximal inspiration in 1 second during a forced maneuver. FEV_1/FVC ratios below 75% are abnormal and characteristic of the obstructive lung diseases.

If **asthma** is suspected on clinical grounds but initial PFTs are normal, two additional assessments can be made. The tests can be repeated after administration of a bronchodilator; a significant increase (15%) over the baseline values suggests reversible airway obstruction. If there is no improvement after administration of bronchodilators and asthma is still suspected, then bronchoprovocation testing can be done. In this test, the patient inhales a substance, such as methacholine, that causes a subclinical but easily detectable fall in airflow in asthmatic patients.

In evaluating the patient with dyspnea, normal PFTs (no response to bronchodilators and no fall in airflow in response to a methacholine challenge) mean that significant pulmonary pathology is unlikely, and another cause of dyspnea should be sought. A cardiac evaluation may be indicated, as shortness of breath can be a manifestation of angina, valvular heart disease, or congestive heart failure. If no cardiac or pulmonary disease is demonstrated, dyspnea may be occurring on the basis of deconditioning, or even anxiety, though this diagnosis should not be made until all other diagnoses have been excluded.

Despite the present patient's history of firefighting and exposure to multiple inhalants, no abnormalities were demonstrated by routine PFTs. A nonpulmonary cause of dyspnea is being sought in this case.

Clinical Pearls

1. Most clinicians require a 12–15% increase in FEV_1 from the pre-drug baseline to define a significant bronchodilator response.

2. The FEV_1 is the most commonly assessed parameter for quantifying bronchodilator effects.

3. Exercise and/or bronchoprovocation testing should be used to determine the presence of exercise-induced bronchospasm and to evaluate the effectiveness of therapeutic regimens.

REFERENCES

1. Eliasson AH, Phillips YY, Rajagopal KR, et al. Sensitivity and specificity of bronchial provocation testing: An evaluation of four techniques in exercise induced bronchospasm. Chest 1992;102:347–355.
2. American Thoracic Society. Lung function testing: Selection of reference values and interpretive strategies. Am Rev Respir Dis 1991;144:1202–1218.
3. Light RW, Conrad SA, George RB. The one best test for evaluating the effects of bronchodilator therapy. Chest 1977;72:512–516.

PATIENT 45

A 7-month-old boy with fever and cough

A 7-month-old boy with a fever and dry cough was brought to the emergency department by his mother. The child was well until one day prior when he developed rhinorrhea and a barking cough. He was the product of a full-term gestation and an uncomplicated delivery, and he had been healthy until the present illness.

Physical Examination: Temperature 103°; pulse 158; respirations 32. Chest: harsh vesicular bilateral breath sounds with scattered rhonchi; inspiratory stridor noted. Cardiac: tachycardic. Abdomen: without masses. Extremities: no cyanosis. Neurologic: normal.

Laboratory Findings: SaO_2 (room air): 94%. Soft-tissue neck radiograph: see below.

Question: What is the cause of the patient's cough?

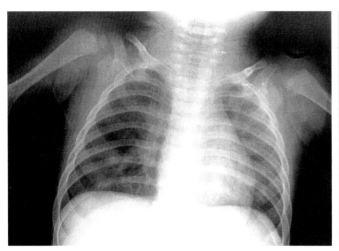 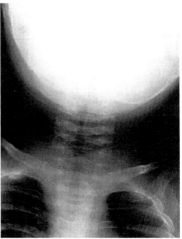

Diagnosis: Croup (laryngotracheobronchitis).

Discussion: Croup (laryngotracheobronchitis) is a syndrome produced by acute infection of the upper air passages and most commonly is seen in children under 3 years of age. It is caused primarily by the parainfluenza and influenza viruses, although respiratory syncytial virus (RSV) and *Mycoplasma pneumoniae* are sometimes implicated. The illness has its greatest frequency in late fall and early winter, but it also follows the epidemic peaks of its viral etiologies. Pathophysiology is primarily one of circumferential mucosal inflammation in the subglottic larynx and trachea, with variable involvement and spasm of the vocal cords. The resultant **subglottic narrowing** causes various degrees of upper airway obstruction. Anteroposterior neck radiographs can demonstrate this narrowing—the subglottic region exhibits a sharply sloped appearance, termed the steeple sign, rather than a shoulder-like silhouette. Infants, whose tracheas are characteristically small, can be significantly compromised by this narrowing of the upper airway.

The child with croup frequently presents with a prodrome of runny nose and low-grade fever after having been ill for several days. A barking or brassy cough with or without stridor and hoarseness is the clinical hallmark. The patient may have suprasternal and substernal retractions and nasal flaring that, along with the stridor, worsen with agitation. Oxygen saturation may be decreased, and in severe cases of obstruction, the $PaCO_2$ may be elevated.

One of the critical decisions in the differential diagnosis of a patient, especially a child, who presents to the emergency ward with shortness of breath and a cough is whether the patient has croup or the potentially more life-threatening **epiglottitis**. Epiglottitis, usually caused by the bacterium *Haemophilus influenzae*, tends to occur in children aged 2–6 years, whereas croup peaks in the first 2 years of life. Additionally, onset of epiglottitis is more sudden, the cough usually is non-barking, and the voice may be muffled. A lateral neck radiograph shows an enlarged epiglottis, and patients typically are intubated to protect against sudden intractable airway obstruction that can lead to asphyxiation. In contrast, croup patients rarely require intubation.

Mild cases of croup, in which patients are stridorous but playful and able to exchange air with only slightly increased effort, are treated supportively with cool aerosol. When respiratory effort and irritability increase, and the child is unable to play or eat comfortably, hospitalization is indicated. Care is based largely on manifestation of symptoms and focuses on careful monitoring for progressive respiratory compromise. Regular assessment of the patient's respiratory rate, degree of retractions, mental status, oxygen saturation, and air exchange is essential. Oxygen therapy is provided, as most children will be somewhat hypoxic. A recent study indicated that the use of steroids may improve outcome and reduce relapse. Aerosolized racemic epinephrine can relieve airway obstruction by inducing local vasoconstriction, and some studies have indicated that this therapy can reduce the need for intubation. The potential for return of the original, or even worsened (rebound) respiratory distress several hours after therapy mandates prolonged observation of the child following the treatment.

The present patient responded to treatment with acetaminophen, humidified oxygen, and aerosolized racemic epinephrine and was discharged 4 days after admission.

Clinical Pearls

1. Approximately 3–5% of all children have at least one episode of viral croup; < 10% of them need hospitalization, and ≤ 2% of those admitted require mechanical ventilation.

2. Patients with croup present with a barking cough, whereas patients with epiglottitis may exhibit a muffled voice and drooling.

3. A lateral neck radiograph should be obtained in patients with suspected croup or epiglottitis. In croup the radiograph may demonstrate subglottic narrowing, and in epiglottitis it shows an enlarged epiglottis.

REFERENCES

1. Tong MC, Chu MC, Leighton SE, van Hasselt CA. Adult croup. Chest 1996;109:1659–1662.
2. Cruz MN, Stewart G, Rosenberg N. Use of dexamethasone in the outpatient management of acute laryngotracheitis. Pediatrics 1995;96:220–223.
3. De Boeck K. Croup: A review. Eur J Pediatr 1995;154:432–436.
4. Harper MB. Pediatric infectious disease emergencies. Curr Opin Pediatr 1995;7:302–308.
5. Schroeder LL, Knapp JF. Recognition and emergency management of infectious causes of upper airway obstruction in children. Semin Respir Infect 1995;10:21–30.
6. Cressman WR, Myer CM 3rd. Diagnosis and management of croup and epiglottitis. Pediatr Clin North Am 1994;42:265–276.

PATIENT 46

A 30-year-old man with weakness, dizziness, and vomiting for 2 days

A 30-year-old man was brought to the emergency department complaining of generalized malaise, dizziness, and vomiting for 2 days. His medical history included insulin-dependent diabetes mellitus over the last 16 years, for which he was taking insulin.

Physical Examination: Temperature 98.2°; pulse 108; respirations 18; blood pressure 130/80. Chest: clear. Cardiac: tachycardic. Abdomen: diminished bowel sounds. Extremities: no cyanosis, clubbing, or edema. Neurologic: lethargic but oriented, nonfocal.

Laboratory Findings: WBC 9420/µl, Hct 43.8%. K^+ 3.2 mEq/L. Glucose 541 mg/dl, anion gap 27 mEq/L, serum ketones positive. ABG (room air): pH 7.23, pCO_2 29 mmHg, pO_2 93 mmHg, HCO_3^- 12 mEq/L, SaO_2 98%. Chest radiograph: see below.

Questions: What is the most likely diagnosis in this patient? What are the general considerations in the treatment of this patient?

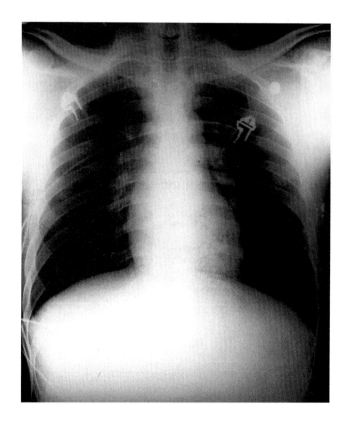

Diagnosis: Diabetic ketoacidosis.

Discussion: Diabetes mellitus (DM) is a common condition affecting more than 12 million Americans. Most patients with DM have so-called type II diabetes, sometimes referred to as adult onset, non–ketosis-prone, or non–insulin-requiring diabetes. Type II is largely believed to be a syndrome of insulin resistance related to obesity. A smaller percentage of patients have type I diabetes, also called juvenile onset, ketosis-prone, or insulin-requiring diabetes. Type I, caused by a lack of insulin, may be due to an auto-immune mediated destruction of pancreatic islet cells.

Although the chronic complications of DM, such as renal failure, retinopathy, neuropathy, and accelerated atherosclerosis, occur in both type I and type II (and, in fact, because more individuals have type II DM, it accounts for more kidney and eye disease than does type I), the acute complications of the two syndromes differ somewhat. Patients with type II DM are prone to develop hyperosmolar, non-ketotic coma marked by severe hyperglycemia (glucose levels of greater than 1000 mg/dl are not unusual) without metabolic acidosis. Patients with type I DM are prone to develop diabetic ketoacidosis (DKA) marked by less severe hyperglycemia but significant **metabolic acidosis**; hence the name of the syndrome.

DKA is a potentially life-threatening complication of diabetes. In its pure form, it is manifested by ketoacidosis and modest hyperglycemia without significant hyperosmolality. DKA occurs when insulin levels are too low to oppose the effects of excessive concentrations of glucagon, catecholamines, cortisol, and growth hormone that are secreted in response to a variety of stressors. Infection is the most common precipitant of DKA, but other triggers include myocardial infarction, hyperthyroidism, and trauma. Non-compliance with insulin therapy and other treatment errors account for approximately 25% of cases of DKA.

Patients with advanced DKA typically present with signs and symptoms that develop rapidly over fewer than 24 hours. The hallmark symptoms are **polyuria** and **polydipsia**, and the physical exam may reveal signs associated with hypovolemia, such as tachycardia and hypotension. Deep respirations (Kussmaul respirations) are often seen, and with severe acidosis the patient may be lethargic. The laboratory examination usually shows a blood glucose concentration greater than 250 mg/dl, and an anion-gap metabolic acidosis invariably is present. Plasma ketone bodies can be detected and quantitated; the three ketone bodies formed in DKA are beta-hydroxybutarate, acetoacetate, and acetone. The anion gap is characteristically increased as a result of the accumulation of beta-hydroxybutarate and acetoacetate. In addition, patients with DKA are usually markedly dehydrated, with total body water deficits of 100 ml/kg and sodium deficits of up to 7–10 mEq/L per kg of body weight. The dehydration is caused by free water losses resulting from the osmotic diuresis caused by hyperglycemia. Blood urea nitrogen is usually elevated out of proportion to the creatinine because of dehydration and prerenal azotemia.

The fundamentals of DKA treatment may be divided into the following categories: general therapeutic measures, fluids, insulin, potassium, and alkali. Of these, hydration is the mainstay of therapy for DKA and independently may cause a 20% or greater reduction in blood glucose levels by improving renal perfusion. Equally important is the administration of a continuous intravenous infusion of regular insulin, which is needed to reverse the acidosis. Insulin should be continued until serum ketones disappear, even if this means administering glucose to prevent hypoglycemia. Although the serum potassium level is usually normal or high in DKA, it invariably falls with rehydration and should be followed closely.

Bicarbonate administration remains somewhat controversial. Most patients respond quickly to fluid and insulin, and bicarbonate therapy is not needed. If the pH is less than 7.0 and/or if the patient presents with coexistent lactic acidosis and severe hyperkalemia, bicarbonate may be given, but pH and electrolytes should be checked soon after.

The present patient was admitted to the medical intensive care unit; after 36 hours, his glucose returned to 108 mg/dl. He was transferred to a general medical floor and was discharged on day 7 with specific nutritional and medication compliance instructions.

Clinical Pearls

1. Disorders of glucose metabolism are common endocrine problems, with diabetes mellitus alone afflicting at least 5% of the population in the United States.

2. Hyperglycemia, hyperketonemia, and acidosis are the hallmarks of diabetic ketoacidosis, developing in patients with either an absolute or relative insulin deficiency.

3. The administration of bicarbonate in diabetic ketoacidosis remains controversial; however, accepted practice allows its administration if the pH is less than 7.0 or in the presence of coexistent lactic acidosis and severe hyperkalemia.

REFERENCES

1. Umpierrez GE, Khajavi M, Kitabchi AE. Review: Diabetic ketoacidosis and hyperglycemic hyperosmolar nonketotic syndrome. Am J Med Sci 1996;311:225–233.
2. Okuda Y, Adrogue HJ, Field JB, et al. Counterproductive effects of sodium bicarbonate in diabetic ketoacidosis. J Clin Endocrinol Metab 1996;81:314–320.
3. Lebovitz HE. Diabetic ketoacidosis. Lancet 1995;345:767–772.
4. Paulson WD, Gadallah MF. Diagnosis of mixed acid–base disorders in diabetic ketoacidosis. Amer J Med Sci 1993;306: 295–300.

PATIENT 47

A 38-year-old man with shortness of breath and productive cough with hemoptysis

A 38-year-old man was brought to the emergency department with shortness of breath, severe body pain, and a cough productive of blood. Medical history included tracheostomy for upper airway obstruction.

Physical Examination: Temperature 99.1°; pulse 104; respirations 20; blood pressure 100/70. HEENT: flattened bridge of nose. Chest: scattered rhonchi. Cardiac: regular rhythm without murmurs or rubs. Abdomen: without masses or organomegaly. Extremities: no cyanosis, clubbing, or edema. Neurologic: alert, nonfocal.

Laboratory Findings: WBC 5420/μl, Hct 32.9%, ESR 52 mm/hr. Glucose 85 mg/dl, BUN 23 mg/dl, Cr 2.1 mg/dl. ABG (room air): pH 7.47, pCO_2 34 mmHg, pO_2 71 mmHg. HCO_3^- 25 mEq/L. SaO_2 95%. Chest radiograph (see below): bilateral nodular opacities.

Question: Are the upper airway obstruction and pulmonary nodules related processes?

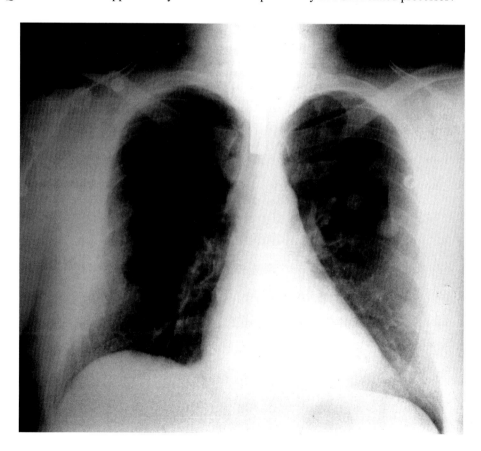

Diagnosis: Wegener's granulomatosis.

Discussion: Wegener's granulomatosis (WG) is a multisystem pathologic entity of unknown etiology characterized by granulomatous vasculitis predominantly involving the upper and lower respiratory tracts and, classically, the kidneys. In its limited form, Wegener's granulomatosis spares the kidneys, but in the full-blown syndrome eyes, heart, skin, ears, and central and peripheral nervous systems can be involved.

Respiratory tract involvement can begin at the nose and extend to the alveolar spaces. **Sinusitis** and **rhinitis** frequently are presenting complaints, though these nonspecific symptoms generally do not prompt a diagnostic evaluation for WG. Nasal involvement can range from rhinitis and epistaxis to destruction of the nasal septal cartilage, resulting in saddle-nose deformity as seen in this patient. Upper airway lesions include laryngeal masses that may mimic laryngeal carcinoma.

However, the most typical respiratory involvement is seen in the **pulmonary parenchyma**, and virtually no patient with WG is without some pulmonary symptoms. Complaints include breathlessness, cough, and hemoptysis representing alveolar hemorrhage. Chest radiographs can show infiltrates, masses, or nodules which may cavitate; these abnormalities may or may not be bilateral. Pulmonary function tests are typically non-diagnostic, though an obstructive pattern may be detected in later disease.

WG is diagnosed when a characteristic clinical syndrome is accompanied by typical pathologic features on a biopsy specimen. Lung biopsies generally reveal necrosis with a granulomatous inflammation characterized by the presence of neutrophils, eosinophils, histiocytes, and vasculitis. Recently there has been a great deal written about the usefulness of antineutrophil cytoplasm antibodies (C-ANCA) in the diagnosis of WG. It has been suggested by some that in the proper clinical setting, a high titer C-ANCA is diagnostic of WG and obviates the need for a tissue biopsy. More recent data suggest that the test may not be as sensitive as initially thought, and an open lung biopsy remains the gold standard for diagnosis. The C-ANCA test does not seem sensitive enough to guide decisions about therapy. WG can be differentiated from allergic granulomatous angiitis (Churg-Strauss syndrome) by the absence of asthma and of peripheral eosinophilia in WG patients.

For many years, WG carried a dismal prognosis, and treatment with corticosteroids was marginally effective. Most patients treated with steroids died of their disease in a relatively short period of time after diagnosis. The outlook for these patients has dramatically improved due to treatment with **cyclophosphamide**. Treatment is begun with a dose of 1–2 mg/kg/day and generally is continued for a year after clinical improvement, with or without the addition of steroids. This approach to treatment should achieve remission in up to 90% of patients. Recent studies indicate that treatment with trimethoprim-sulfamethoxazole may help prevent relapse once remission has been achieved.

The present patient's open lung biopsy revealed granulomatous inflammation. His C-ANCA was positive, and a diagnosis of WG was made. His previous upper airway obstruction likely represented a bout of limited WG. He was treated with oral cyclophosphamide and prednisolone and was discharged from the hospital 6 days after admission on this therapeutic regimen.

Clinical Pearls

1. The prognosis of Wegener's granulomatosis (WG) treated with cyclophosphamide is excellent, with marked improvement seen in approximately 90% of patients and complete remission in 75% of patients.

2. Elevated titers of antineutrophil cytoplasm antibodies (C-ANCA) strongly support the diagnosis of WG; however, a negative C-ANCA does not rule out the diagnosis.

3. WG should be included in the differential diagnosis of upper airway obstruction, even in the absence of pulmonary parenchymal lesions.

REFERENCES

1. Edgar JD. The clinical utility of ANCA positivity. Ann Rheum Dis 1996;55:494–496.
2. Stegeman CA, Cohen Tervaert JW, de Jong PE, Kallengerg CG. Trimethoprim-sulfamethoxazole (co-trimoxazole) for the prevention of relapses of Wegener's granulomatosis. N Engl J Med 1996;335:16–20.
3. Schultz DR, Tozman EC. Antineutrophil cytoplasmic antibodies: Major autoantigens, pathophysiology, and disease associations. Semin Arthritis Rheum 1995;25:143–159.
4. Rao JK, Allen NB, Feussner JR, Weinberger M. A prospective study of antineutrophil cytoplasmic antibody (c-ANCA) and clinical criteria in diagnosing Wegener's granulomatosis. Lancet 1995;346:926–931.
5. Chapman PT, O'Donnell JL. Respiratory failure in Wegener's granulomatosis: Response to pulse intravenous methylprednisolone and cyclophosphamide. J. Rheumatol 1993;20:504–506.

PATIENT 48

A 64-year-old woman with shortness of breath and fatigue for 2 days

A 64-year-old woman presented to the emergency department complaining of shortness of breath and fatigue for 2 days. Her medical history included lung cancer diagnosed 3 years earlier for which she underwent a left apical lobectomy. Her disease recurred and she was treated with chemotherapy and pleurodesis for a malignant pleural effusion. Two months prior to the current admission a CT scan of the head revealed metastasis to the brain, and 1 month ago a CT scan of the abdomen revealed metastasis to the liver. The patient denied any smoking history.

Physical Examination: Temperature 98.6°; pulse 104; respirations 26; blood pressure 130/80. Chest: bilateral vesicular breath sounds, markedly diminished breath sounds on the left. Cardiac: regular rhythm without murmurs. Abdomen: hepatomegaly. Extremities: no cyanosis; lower extremities revealed 2$^+$ pitting edema. Neurologic: alert and oriented.

Laboratory Findings: WBC 12,000/μl, Hct 38%. Na$^+$ 137 mEq/L, K$^+$ 4.5 mEq/L, CL$^-$ 87 mEq/L, HCO$_3^-$ 33 mEq/L. ALK PHOS 154 U/L, GGT 289 IU/L, LDH 1146 IU/L. ABG (room air): pH 7.46, pCO$_2$ 44 mmHg, pO$_2$ 59 mmHg, HCO$_3^-$ 30 mEq/L, SaO$_2$ 91%. Chest radiograph (see below): left apical lobectomy.

Question: What condition most likely explains the patient's clinical presentation?

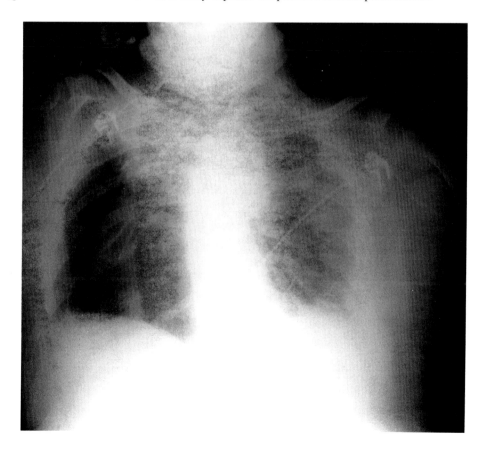

Diagnosis: Respiratory failure due to adenocarcinoma of the lung.

Discussion: Lung cancer, also called bronchogenic carcinoma, is the leading cause of cancer deaths in the United States among both men and women. Each year there are more than 175,000 new cases of lung cancer in the U.S., and more than 150,000 persons die. Approximately 85% of lung cancer cases are related directly to tobacco use, and the remainder are linked to second-hand smoke (environmental tobacco smoke) and other toxins such as radon. Lung cancer mortality rates fell slightly in 1995, but probably due to a decrease in the incidence of smoking rather than to substantial improvements in lung cancer therapy.

Four major cell types make up 95% of all primary lung neoplasms: squamous or epidermoid carcinoma, adenocarcinoma, large cell carcinoma, and small cell (oat cell) carcinoma. The various cell types have different natural histories and responses to therapy, so a correct histologic diagnosis is essential to proper treatment. Major treatment decisions are based on the crucial distinction between **histologic classification** of a tumor as a small cell carcinoma (SCC) or as one of the non-small cell carcinoma (NSCC) varieties (which include epidermoid, adenocarcinoma, large cell carcinoma, and mixed versions).

Ninety percent of patients with lung cancer of all histologic types are cigarette smokers, while the rare nonsmoking patient who develops lung cancer usually has adenocarcinoma. In nonsmokers with adenocarcinoma involving the lung, the possibility of other primary sites should be considered.

Cancer of the lung develops insidiously, often giving little or no warning of its presence. Because its symptoms are similar to those associated with smoking and chronic bronchitis, they are often disregarded. Lung cancers produce their local effects by irritation and obstruction of the airways and invasion of the mediastinum and pleural space. The earliest symptoms include chronic cough, shortness of breath, and wheezing due to airway irritation and obstruction. Hemoptysis occurs when the lesion erodes blood vessels. Pain receptors in the chest are limited to the parietal pleura, mediastinum, larger blood vessels, and peribronchial afferent vagal fibers; thus, lung cancers usually are painless until far advanced. Dull, intermittent, poorly localized retrosternal pain is common in tumors that involve the mediastinum. Pain becomes persistent, localized, and more severe when the disease invades the pleura.

Diagnosis of lung cancer is usually triggered by a chest radiograph demonstrating a suspicious lesion, followed by a transbronchial or transthoracic lung biopsy. Once a cancer has been diagnosed, treatment decisions are based on histologic type and stage. SCC virtually is never operated on. If SCC is limited to one hemithorax and can be contained within a radiation port, a combination of chemotherapy and radiation therapy is given. If the disease extends beyond a hemithorax, chemotherapy alone is given. Despite treatment, median survival for patients with SCC is only about 1 year.

NSCC is treated surgically whenever possible; if the disease is in stages I (tumor alone) or II (disease not spread beyond hilar lymph nodes), resection is the best approach. Once the disease has involved the mediastinal lymph nodes, prognosis is dismal. Unfortunately, the vast majority of lung cancer patients present with advanced disease, and 5-year survival for all patients with lung cancer is only about 13%.

The best way to prevent lung cancer deaths is to abstain from tobacco use. Early detection and diagnosis through yearly screening chest radiographs and sputum cytologic examination have not been demonstrated to improve overall outcome in lung cancer; therefore, routine chest radiographs in smokers generally are not recommended. Recently, however, interest in targeting patients for cancer surveillance if they are at especially high risk (e.g., patients with chronic obstructive pulmonary disease) has reemerged.

The present patient was treated with palliative radiation therapy, chemotherapy, oxygen, aminophylline, prednisolone, and albuterol metered-dose inhaler. Because of the advanced stage of carcinoma, arrangements were made for admission to a hospice.

Clinical Pearls

1. Lung cancer is the leading cause of cancer deaths in the United States among both men and women, and the vast majority of lung cancers are related directly to cigarette smoking.

2. The major histologic subdivisions of lung cancer are small cell cancer and non-small sell cancer. The latter includes adenocarcinoma, squamous cell carcinoma, and large cell carcinoma.

3. Screening chest radiographs in smokers have not been demonstrated to improve overall outcome in lung cancer and are not recommended on a routine basis. High-risk patients, wuch as those with chronic obstructive pulmonary disease, may benefit from periodic chest radiographs.

REFERENCES

1. Hoffmann D, Rivenson A, Hecht SS. The biological significance of tobacco-specific N-nitrosamines: Smoking and adenocarcinoma of the lung. Crit Rev Toxicol 1996;26:199–211.
2. Edelman MJ, Gandara DR, Roach M 3rd, Benfield JR. Multimodality therapy in stage III non-small cell lung cancer. Ann Thorac Surg 1996;61(5):1564–1572.
3. Dev D, Capewell S, Sankaran R, et al. Adenocarcinoma of the lung: Clinical features and survival. Respir Med 1996; 90:333–337.
4. Reynolds P, Fontham ET. Passive smoking and lung cancer. Ann Med 1995;27:633–640.
5. Wynder EL, Muscat JE. The changing epidemiology of smoking and lung cancer histology. Environ Health Perspect 1995; 103(Suppl 8):143–148.
6. Jett JR. Current treatment of unresectable lung cancer. Mayo Clin Proc 1993;68:603–611.

PATIENT 49

A 25-year-old woman with right-sided chest pain and difficulty breathing

A 25-year-old woman was brought to the emergency department complaining of right-sided chest pain, worse with inspiration, and dyspnea for 1 day. She had been well, but became symptomatic while driving home from work. She had smoked cigarettes for five years.

Physical Examination: Temperature 98.7°; pulse 80; respirations 24; blood pressure 122/76. Chest: diminished breath sounds over the left lung. Cardiac: without murmurs or rubs. Abdomen: without masses or organomegaly. Neurologic: alert, nonfocal.

Laboratory Findings: WBC 9300/μl, Hct 45%. Glucose 88 mg/dl. ABG (room air): pH 7.42, pCO_2 29 mmHg, pO_2 79 mmHg, HCO_3^- 16 mEq/L, SaO_2 96%. Chest radiograph: see below.

Question: What therapy should be instituted?

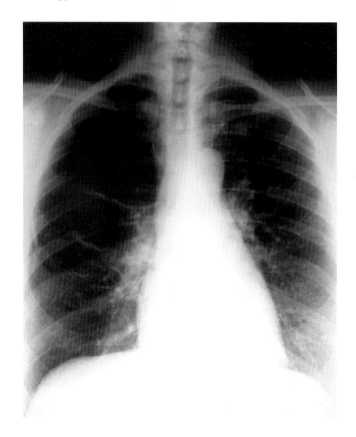

Diagnosis: Spontaneous pneumothorax.

Discussion: Pneumothorax (PTX) is the presence of air in the pleural space. Spontaneous PTX, which occurs without antecedent trauma to the thorax, is considered primary when it occurs in individuals *without* known underlying lung disease, and secondary when it occurs in individuals *with* underlying lung disease. The differential diagnosis of spontaneous PTX includes rupture of **subpleural blebs**, which occur in patients with emphysema, including disease caused by alpha-1-antitrypsin deficiency; Marfan's syndrome and other connective tissue disorders; diseases such as eosinophilic granuloma, lymphangioleiomyomatosis (which occurs only in women), and tuberous sclerosis (with pathology almost identical to lymphangioleiomyomatosis); and chronic and severe lung diseases such as sarcoidosis and cystic fibrosis.

Subpleural blebs also occur in smokers, often in the absence of overt emphysema. Overall, primary spontaneous PTX is believed to result most commonly from rupture of a subpleural emphysematous bleb. There is a strong association between smoking and the development of primary spontaneous PTX. Moreover, interestingly, these patients tend to be taller and thinner than average.

The main physiologic consequences of PTX are a decrease in vital capacity and a decrease in arterial pO_2 due to ventilation/perfusion abnormalities and shunting. Decreased vital capacity in the patient with primary spontaneous PTX usually is well tolerated, and hypoxemia usually is not severe. If the lung function of the patient is compromised before PTX occurs, the decrease in vital capacity may lead to respiratory insufficiency, alveolar hypoventilation, and respiratory failure.

The diagnosis of PTX typically is suggested by the clinical history and the physical examination. The diagnosis is established by demonstrating a pleural line and the absence of lung markings on the chest radiograph. CT scans of the chest can be extremely helpful in defining any underlying lung disease as well as demonstrating the presence and location of subpleural blebs.

Observation, administration of supplemental oxygen, simple aspiration, and tube thoracostomy are available therapeutic options. With no intervention, only about 1% of the volume of the PTX is reabsorbed each day. Some have advocated the use of 100% oxygen breathing based on the theory that it creates a gradient for nitrogen and allows the air that has leaked into the pleural space to be reabsorbed more rapidly. There is little empiric data to prove the value of this approach. For a substantial PTX, tube thoracostomy seems to be the most effective therapeutic option. Small tubes appear to be sufficient and should be considered if simple aspiration is unsuccessful. Rarely, following re-expansion of the collapsed lung, unilateral or bilateral pulmonary edema occurs. This complication arises about 1% of the time.

Generally, if no underlying lung disease is found, no further therapy is indicated after an *initial* spontaneous PTX, and the patient simply is observed. For *recurrent* PTX, pleurodesis, stapling or resection of blebs, and other procedures are employed. Though open thoracotomy has been the standard approach to definitive treatment for recurrent PTX, video-assisted thoracoscopic surgery rapidly has come into use as an alternative, less morbid approach.

The present patient underwent tube thoracostomy which resulted in lung re-expansion. The chest tube was removed 2 days after insertion and the patient was discharged 48 hours later without event.

Clinical Pearls

1. In spontaneous pneumothorax (PTX), only about 1% of the volume of the PTX is re-absorbed every 24 hours, so that aspiration or evacuation is necessary in most cases.

2. 100% oxygen breathing may increase the rate of absorption of air in the pleural space by creating a gradient for nitrogen.

3. Patients with primary spontaneous PTX initially should be managed with simple aspiration of the pleural air. If simple aspiration is unsuccessful, then tube thoracostomy should be performed. Recurrent pneumothorax generally is an indication for surgical intervention.

REFERENCES

1. Rozenman J, Yellin A, Simansky DA, Shiner RJ. Re-expansion pulmonary edema following spontaneous pneumothorax. Respir Med 1996;90:235–238.
2. Mouroux J, Elkaim D, Padovani B, et al. Video-assisted thoracoscopic treatment of spontaneous pneumothorax: Technique and results of 100 cases. J Thorac Cardiovasc Surg 1996;112:385–391.
3. Berkman N, Bloom A, Cohen P, et al. Bilateral spontaneous pneumothorax as the presenting feature in lymphangioleiomy-omatosis. Respir Med 1995;89:381–383.
4. Andrivet P, Djedaini K, Teboul JL, et al. Spontaneous pneumothorax: Comparison of thoracic drainage vs immediate or delayed needle aspiration. Chest 1995;108:335–339.

PATIENT 50

A 16-month-old girl with fever, cough, and difficulty breathing

A 16-month-old girl was brought to the emergency department with fever of 2-weeks' duration and subsequent onset of a cough and severe difficulty breathing. Two days prior her pediatrician had diagnosed pharyngitis and otitis media and prescribed amoxicillin.

Physical Examination: Temperature 102.5°; pulse 152; respirations 48; blood pressure 82/48. General: obvious respiratory distress. HEENT: erythematous, bulging left tympanic membrane. Chest: inspiratory stridor heard over the trachea. Cardiac: tachycardic. Abdomen: without organomegaly. Extremities: cyanosis. Neurologic: lethargic.

Laboratory Findings: SpO_2 (room air): 80%. Chest radiograph: see below.

Hospital Course: In the emergency department, the patient was given dexamethasone 4 mg and ceftriaxone 250 mg IV. Aerosolized racemic epinephrine was provided via small volume nebulizer. The patient did not respond and was intubated for respiratory distress. She was then transferred to the intensive care unit where she was stabilized and placed on a BEAR CUB infant ventilator with the following settings: PIP 25 cm H_2O, f = 18, CMV/IMV, flow 8 L/min, FiO_2 .35, with 5 cm H_2O PEEP.

Question: What is the cause of the respiratory distress in this patient?

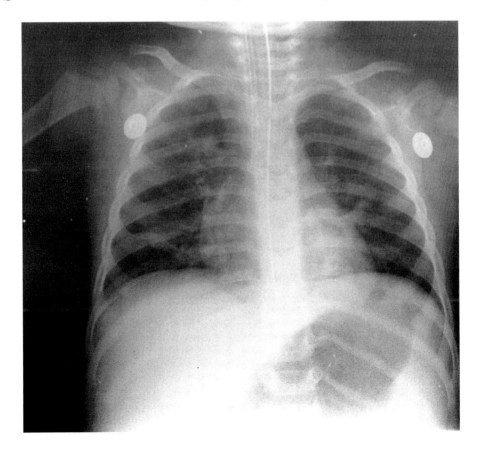

Diagnosis: Acute epiglottitis.

Discussion: Acute epiglottitis is a true medical emergency. It results from bacterial invasion of the soft tissues of the larynx, which leads to sudden, marked swelling of the epiglottis and surrounding tissues and rapid closing of the glottic opening. The most common causative organism is *Haemophilus influenzae*, type B. Much less frequently, staphylococci and streptococci cause the disorder. Historically, epiglottitis has been a disease of early childhood that rarely recurs. The incidence and age distribution of epiglottitis is changing, however, because of the recent widespread use of the *H. influenzae* type B vaccine.

The child with epiglottitis classically presents with a sudden development of high fever, severe sore throat, difficulty swallowing, hoarse or abnormal voice, drooling, and stridor. Patients frequently demonstrate flaring of the alae nasae, retraction of the intercostal muscles, and dyspnea. They maintain an upright position, and lean forward with the neck extended (sniffing position) in an attempt to keep the epiglottis from obstructing the glottis. A major point of differential diagnosis is distinguishing **croup** (laryngotracheitis) from epiglottitis. Croup is seen in younger children and presents with a somewhat insidious onset and a brassier cough. Epiglottitis presents with acute onset, toxic appearance, and a non-barking cough.

Since manipulation or agitation of the child with epiglottitis can trigger complete obstruction of the upper airway, it is imperative that the evaluation, diagnosis, and therapeutic intervention center on maintaining a calm, nonthreatening atmosphere. Until **controlled intubation** can be accomplished, there should be no attempts made to visualize the laryngeal area, draw blood, or lay the child flat for an examination. The patient should be permitted to sit upright, left in the parent's arms, and treated with blow-by oxygen when needed. *At no time should a child with suspected epiglottitis be left unattended by medical personnel.* This is particularly true when the child is sent for lateral neck radiographs, which usually demonstrate the swollen epiglottis characteristic of the syndrome.

Since the upper airway structures are markedly swollen in the child with epiglottitis, an endotracheal tube one size smaller than that indicated by the patient's age and size should be used. Once in place, it should remain so for 12–48 hours until the inflamed tissue shrinks in response to antibiotic therapy and steroids. Close supervision, arm restraints, and pharmacologic sedation and paralysis can prevent attempts at self-extubation. Extubation is considered when signs of infection such as fever diminish or direct visualization of the epiglottis reveals that adequate tissue shrinkage has occurred.

The present patient was supported with mechanical ventilation and treated with antibiotics. By the third day following admission the epiglottic swelling had dissipated to permit extubation. She was discharged on cefaclor seven days following admission.

Clinical Pearls

1. *Haemophilus influenzae* is the most common causative organism of epiglottitis in children younger than 6 years of age.

2. Because the tip of the laryngoscope blade is placed in the vallecula to avoid direct contact with the epiglottis, curved laryngoscope blades are the blades of choice for intubation in epiglottitis.

3. Endotracheal tube selection should be one size smaller than that indicated by the patient's age and size in order to minimize aggravation of swollen tissue during intubation.

REFERENCES
1. Carey MJ. Epiglottitis in adults. Am J Emerg Med 1996;14:421–442.
2. Young N, Finn A, Powell C. Group B Streptococcal epiglottitis. Pediatr Infect Dis J 1996;15:95–96.
3. Gilbert GL, Johnson PD, Clements DA. Clinical manifestations and outcome of *Haemophilus influenzae* type B. J Paediatr Child Health 1995;31:99–104.
4. Gonzalez Valdepena H, Wald ER, Rose E, et al. Epiglottitis and *Haemophilus influenzae* immunization: The Pittsburgh experience—a five-year review. Pediatrics 1995;96:424–427.
5. Schroeder LL, Knapp JF. Recognition and emergency management of infectious causes of upper airway obstruction in children. Semin Respir Infect 1995;10:21–30.

PATIENT 51

A 20-year-old man with nausea, decreased appetite, epigastric pain, and dark urine for 5 days

A 20-year-old man came to the emergency department complaining of nausea, decreased appetite, epigastric pain, and dark urine of 5 days duration. Importantly, the patient's wife had been diagnosed with hepatitis B 18 months prior. He denied any significant medical history and was taking no medications.

Physical Examination: Temperature 99.3°; pulse 64; respirations 18; blood pressure 120/60. HEENT: icteric sclerae, bilateral cervical adenopathy. Chest: clear. Cardiac: regular rhythm without murmurs. Abdomen: liver palpable three fingerbreadths below the costal margin; stool negative for occult blood. Extremities: no cyanosis, clubbing, or edema. Neurologic: lethargic, but nonfocal.

Laboratory Findings: WBC 4740/μl, Hct 38.5%. Glucose 58 mg/dl, ALK PHOS 228 IU/L, ALT 4993 IU/L, AST 3232 IU/L, GGT 223 IU/L, LDH 4059 IU/L, albumin 3.5 g/dl, total bilirubin 6.7 mg/dl. PT 16.0 sec, PTT 28.4 sec (control 12.1 sec).

Question: How should the patient's lethargy be managed?

Diagnosis: Acute viral hepatitis B.

Discussion: Many varieties of viral infection can cause inflammation in the liver, but among the most important of these are the hepatitis A, B, and C viruses. Hepatitis A, often caused by ingestion of contaminated shellfish, typically causes an acute but self-limited illness that rarely goes on to cause fulminant hepatic failure, chronic hepatitis, or cirrhosis. In fact, hepatitis C (formerly called non-A, non-B hepatitis), whose mode of transmission is still somewhat unclear, probably is the leading cause of cirrhosis in the world. Hepatitis B also is a common cause of acute hepatitis and chronic liver disease. Its usual modes of transmission are sexual contact and the blood-borne route.

The incubation period for hepatitis B is approximately 70–80 days. The prodromal symptoms of acute viral hepatitis are systemic and quite variable. Anorexia, nausea and vomiting, fatigue, malaise, arthralgias, myalgias, headache, photophobia, pharyngitis, cough, and coryza may precede the onset of jaundice by 1–2 weeks. Dark urine and clay-colored stools may be noticed by the patient 1–5 days prior to the onset of clinical jaundice. The diagnosis of hepatitis B is usually straightforward: hepatitis B surface antigen titers are positive in the acute phase of the illness, but then decline as titers of hepatitis B surface antibody become elevated. During the so-called window period, both surface antigen and surface antibody titers may be absent, and the diagnosis may be missed.

The most dangerous complication of acute hepatitis is **fulminant hepatic failure**, in which overwhelming inflammation stops all synthetic and metabolic processes. Patients in this condition have severe coagulopathy which predisposes them to gastrointestinal hemorrhage and other bleeding complications, hepatic encephalopathy, and, frequently, renal failure from the hepatorenal syndrome. Patients with hepatic encephalopathy are prone to aspiration pneumonia that can be overwhelming and fatal. For this reason, if the patient's mental status is significantly depressed, elective intubation is indicated to protect the airway and guard against aspiration.

There is no specific treatment for acute viral hepatitis, and even in cases of fulminant hepatic failure treatment is largely supportive. Although hospitalization may be necessary in clinically severe illness, many patients do not require hospital care.

A special concern for healthcare workers, particularly those working in intensive care units, is **occupational risk** of hepatitis infection. Healthcare workers are frequently exposed to blood, tissue, and body fluids and therefore are at increased risk of contracting viral hepatitis (primarily B). Transmission of hepatitis B infection in healthcare settings appears to occur mostly from patients to staff. Therefore, appropriate protection (universal precautions) should be used by healthcare personnel when performing any procedures likely to expose them to mucous membranes, blood, or body fluids in these patients. Additionally, for preexposure prophylaxis against hepatitis B in settings of frequent exposure, three intramuscular injections of a recombinant hepatitis B vaccine are recommended at 0, 1, and 6 months. Many healthcare organizations will provide titer testing 1–2 weeks after the third dose of vaccine as well as perform follow-up titer testing every 5–6 years to ensure appropriate protection against the virus.

The present patient tested positive for hepatitis B core antibodies and hepatitis B surface antigens. He underwent several days of bed rest, a high calorie diet, and vitamin K therapy. He was discharged home 10 days after admission.

Clinical Pearls

1. At least five different types of hepatitis virus now have been identified and are designated by the letters A–E.

2. Fulminant hepatic failure can complicate infection with both hepatitis B and C, although fulminant hepatitis B is the more common.

3. Patients with fulminant hepatic failure are at risk for hepatic encephalopathy and aspiration pneumonia, and when mental status becomes depressed, consideration should be given to elective intubation to protect the airway.

4. Healthcare workers at risk for exposure to blood and other bodily fluids should receive the recombinant hepatitis B vaccine.

REFERENCES

1. Farci P, Alter HJ, Shimoda A, et al. Hepatitis C virus-associated fulminant hepatic failure. N Engl J Med 1996;335:631–634.
2. Atillasoy E, Berk PD. Fulminant hepatic failure: Pathophysiology, treatment, and survival. Annu Rev Med 1995;46:181–191.
3. Agerton TB, Mahoney FJ, Polish LB, Shapiro CN. Impact of the bloodborne pathogens standard on vaccination of healthcare workers with hepatitis B vaccine. Infect Control Hosp Epidemiol 1995;16:287–291.
4. Hirschman SZ. Current therapeutic approaches to viral hepatitis. Clin Infect Dis 1995;20:741–743.
5. Lettau LA. The A, B, C, D, and E of viral hepatitis: Spelling out the risks for healthcare workers. Infect Control Hosp Epidemiol 1992;13:77–81.

PATIENT 52

An 18-year-old man with fever, headache, and neck pain

An 18-year-old previously healthy man presented to the emergency department complaining of fever, headache, neck pain, and lower back pain of one week's duration.

Physical Examination: Temperature 103°; pulse 68; respirations 18; blood pressure 110/70. HEENT: pharynx clear, tympanic membranes intact and pearly gray. Chest: clear. Cardiac: without murmurs or rubs. Abdomen: without masses or organomegaly. Extremities: no cyanosis or edema. Neurologic: alert and oriented, nuchal rigidity present, positive Kernig's sign, otherwise nonfocal.

Laboratory Findings: WBC 18,700/μl, Hct 47.3%. Glucose 125 mg/dl. Chest radiograph: see below.

Hospital Course: A spinal tap was performed and the patient was started on penicillin, acetaminophen, and codeine. He was then transferred to a medical-surgical floor for further evaluation. CT scan of the head and radiographic evaluation of the cervical spine, lumbar spine, and sacrum were performed.

Questions: What should the initial diagnostic procedure be in this case, and what therapy should be given?

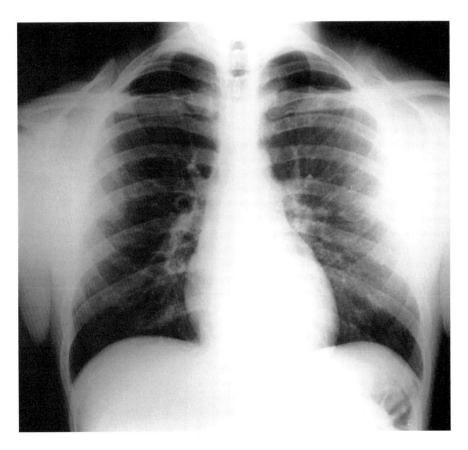

Diagnosis: Acute bacterial meningitis.

Discussion: Bacterial meningitis is a life-threatening infection which requires **prompt diagnosis and treatment** in order to achieve a good outcome without significant morbidity or mortality. The examining physician should focus on performing the indicated diagnostic evaluation in a timely fashion and instituting therapy without delay.

Bacterial meningitis is a common disease worldwide and results in more than 2000 deaths annually in the United States. The relative frequency of isolation of various bacterial species as a cause of meningitis is age related. Gram-negative bacilli (principally *Escherichia coli*, Pseudomonas species, *Listeria monocytogenes*) and group B streptococci are the major causative organisms during the neonatal period. *Haemophilus influenzae* and *Neisseria meningitidis* (meningococcus) are the major causes in children beyond one month of age. Meningitis in adults is due primarily to meningococci and *Streptococcus pneumoniae* (pneumococcus).

The classic clinical presentation of adults with bacterial meningitis includes headache, fever, and meningismus (stiff neck), often with signs of cerebral dysfunction. Nausea, vomiting, rigors, profuse sweats, weakness, myalgias, and photophobia are also common. The meningismus can be subtle or marked, accompanied by Kernig's or Brudzinski's signs. A positive Kernig's sign is recorded when flexion of the knee results in neck pain; for Brudzinski's sign, pain occurs in the back upon flexion of the neck. Cerebral dysfunction is manifested primarily by confusion, delirium, or a declining level of consciousness. Cranial nerve palsies, especially involving cranial nerves IV, VI, and VII, also may be appreciated.

The diagnosis of bacterial meningitis rests with examination of the **cerebrospinal fluid** (CSF) obtained at lumbar puncture. Bacterial meningitis usually is associated with a predominance of polymorphonuclear leukocytes in the CSF and a low glucose level. CSF examination by Gram stain, which may allow presumptive identification of the etiologic agent, should always be performed in suspected cases of meningitis. If the diagnosis is likely, patients should receive emergent empirical **antimicrobial therapy** based on age and underlying disease status—even if no etiologic agent is identified by Gram stain or rapid diagnostic tests. Once the infecting microorganism has been isolated in culture (or identified by other means), antimicrobial therapy is modified for optimal treatment based on susceptibility results.

A key point in the management of the patient with suspected meningitis is the prompt performance of a lumbar puncture and institution of antibiotic therapy. If the lumbar puncture is to be delayed for any reason, a dose of antibiotics should be given. Often, the spinal tap is delayed so that a CT scan of the brain can be performed, but if a careful neurologic exam reveals no focal abnormalities, then usually there is no need to postpone the lumbar puncture. If the presence of penicillin-resistant pneumococcus in the community is high, empiric treatment with penicillin may not be adequate, as CSF penetration of the drug may fail to reach the minimal inhibitory concentration needed to fight the infection.

Direct respiratory abnormalities in meningitis are rare, although depression of consciousness may lead to aspiration pneumonia requiring intubation for airway protection. In addition, pathogens such as *N. meningitidis* may be spread by the airborne route, so isolation is warranted in suspected cases of bacterial meningitis. After 48 hours of therapy, the isolation can be discontinued. Persons coming into close contact with a case of meningococcal meningitis should receive prophylactic antibiotic therapy with rifampin. This includes respiratory therapy personnel who might be involved in intubation or resuscitation.

A lumbar puncture of the present patient demonstrated the presence of polymorphonuclear leukocytes and gram positive diplococci suggestive of pneumococcus. Cultures of CSF eventually grew *S. pneumoniae*. He was treated successfully with penicillin, acetaminophen, and codeine and was discharged on day 10 following admission.

Clinical Pearls

1. Approximately 25,000 cases of meningitis occur annually, of which 70% occur in children under 5 years of age.

2. The cerebrospinal fluid culture is positive in approximately 70–85% of patients with bacterial meningitis.

3. Respiratory isolation during the first 24–48 hours should be considered for all patients suspected of having acute bacterial meningitis. Prophylaxis with rifampin should be taken by all close contacts of a case of meningococcal meningitis.

REFERENCES

1. Tunkel AR, Scheld WM. Acute bacterial meningitis. Lancet 1995;346:1675–1680.
2. Bradley JS, Kaplan SL, Klugman KP, Leggiadro RJ. Consensus: Management of infections in children caused by *Streptococcus pneumoniae* with decreased susceptibility to penicillin. Pediatr Infect Dis J 1995;14:1037–1041.
3. Pfister HW, Feiden W, Einhaupl KM. Spectrum of complications during bacterial meningitis in adults: Results of a prospective clinical study. Arch Neurol 1993;50:575–581.
4. Tunkel AR, Scheld WM. Pathogenesis and pathophysiology of bacterial meningitis. Annu Rev Med 1993;44:103–120.

PATIENT 53

A 42-year-old woman with increasing difficulty breathing over 2 weeks

A 42-year-old woman with a history of asthma noted increasing dyspnea over a two-week period. She had been working for 5 years in a production factory making metal polish, and her medications included theophylline and an albuterol inhaler. She had a long smoking history as well.

Physical Examination: Temperature 98.6°; pulse 80; respirations 22; blood pressure 118/82. Chest: diffuse crackles and bilateral rales at the bases, no wheezing. Cardiac: normal. Abdomen: normal. Extremities: early clubbing. Neurologic: normal.

Laboratory Findings: ABG (room air): pH 7.42, pCO_2 39 mmHg, pO_2 93 mmHg, HCO_3^- 25 mEq/L, SaO_2 97%. PFT: FVC 2.22 L (70% predicted), FEV_1 1.76 L (69% predicted), TLC 4.74 L (92% predicted), DLCO 13 ml/min/mmHg (66% predicted). Chest radiograph: see below.

Question: What causes of dyspnea may be related to the patient's job?

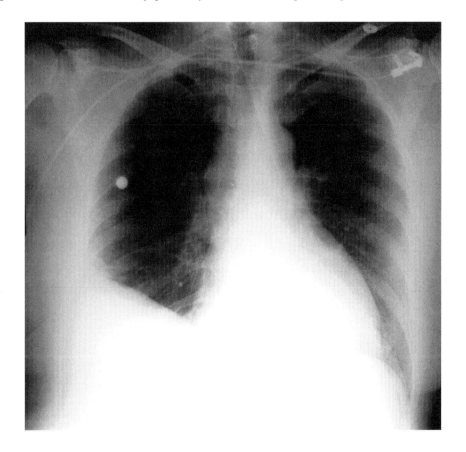

Diagnosis: Acute silicosis.

Discussion: Occupational lung diseases are a major cause of morbidity and mortality in the United States and around the world. Syndromes of asthma, pulmonary fibrosis, the adult respiratory distress syndrome, noncardiogenic pulmonary edema, emphysema, and lung cancer have all been related to one type of **occupational exposure** or another. As evidenced by this list of disorders, the clinical syndromes caused by occupational exposures include many common diseases, so that the clue to the nature of the disorder lies in a careful and thorough history of all current and past jobs held by the patient.

The production of many abrasives, including sandpaper, metal polish, and paint fillers, involves crushing and pulverizing materials that contain **silica dust**, and workers involved in these types of production are at risk for a variety of silica-induced lung diseases. In addition, occupations such as sandblasting, quarrying, glass making, and pottery manufacture also may involve exposure to silica dust and place workers at risk. The major damage to the lungs occurs as the result of inhaling the crystalline form (usually as quartz) of silicon dioxide, known as silica.

There are three syndromes associated with silicosis: a chronic form that typically follows prolonged exposure and is associated with the development of silicotic nodules and focal fibrosis in the hila and upper lobes; an accelerated form following briefer, heavier exposure that is associated with irregular pulmonary fibrosis as well; and an acute form following intense exposure to fine dust of high silica content for periods measured in months rather than years. The acute form can present as alveolar proteinosis in addition to interstitial disease. Moreover, some evidence exists that silicosis is an independent risk factor for lung cancer.

The clinical syndromes associated with silica dust exposure are characterized by **progressive breathlessness**, although occasionally patients are asymptomatic and the diagnosis is suggested by abnormal chest radiographs. Cough also may occur, but symptoms of airway obstruction such as wheezing are uncommon. Clubbing is unusual, and systemic symptoms do not occur.

There are radiographic manifestations of silica-induced lung disease. Small nodules (silicotic nodules) may be apparent on the chest radiograph and are well visualized on CT scans of the lung. The nodules seem to have a predilection for the upper lobes and often have a thin rim of calcification associated with them (egg-shell calcification). As the nodules become heavily fibrotic and contracted, areas of secondary emphysema may form in the lower lung fields. Occasionally, silicosis can be complicated by overwhelming fibrosis (progressive massive fibrosis), and patients with underlying silicosis are at high risk for developing tuberculosis (so-called silicotuberculosis), which may be somewhat difficult to recognize because of the distorted underlying lung architecture.

The Occupational Safety and Health Administration has established that a respiratory protection program must be implemented for all workers at risk for occupational lung disease of any sort, and compliance with these guidelines has reduced job-related lung injury over the past several years. Individual respirator masks should be chosen based on the type of exposure and hazard present in the workplace.

In the present patient, the absence of wheezing led physicians away from a diagnosis of asthma, and a CT scan of the lung demonstrated changes consistent with silicosis. She changed jobs, but lung function deteriorated in subsequent years.

Clinical Pearls

1. The key to diagnosis of any occupational lung disease is a careful and thorough history of all current and prior jobs held by the patient.

2. Silicosis can be associated with a variety of professions, and although distinguishing this syndrome from others on the basis of symptoms alone can be difficult, the presence of wheezing makes the diagnosis unlikely.

3. The exposure limit permitted by the Occupational Safety and Health Administration to crystalline silica is 100 μm/m^3 per airborne dust sample.

REFERENCES

1. Allison AC. Fibrogenic and other biological effects of silica. Curr Top Microbiol Immunol 1996;210:147–158.
2. Murray J, Kielkowski D, Reid P. Occupational disease trends in black South African gold miners: An autopsy-based study. Am J Respir Crit Care Med 1996;153:706–710.
3. Goldsmith DF, Beaumont JJ, Morrin LA, Schenker MB. Respiratory cancer and other chronic disease mortality among silicotics in California. Am J Ind Med 1995;28:459–467.
4. Steenland K, Brown D. Silicosis among gold miners: Exposure–response analyses and risk assessment. Am J Public Health 1995;85:1372–1377.
5. Talini D, Paggiaro PL, Falaschi F, et al. Chest radiography and high resolution computed tomography in the evaluation of workers exposed to silica dust: Relation with functional findings. Occup Environ Med 1995;52:262–267.

PATIENT 54

A 38-year-old man with altered mental status and a high fever

A 38-year-old man was brought to the emergency department in August after he had been found in bed by his family responsive only to painful stimuli. There was no other medical history available.

Physical Examination: Temperature 107.1°; pulse 98; respirations 30; blood pressure 150/96. General physical exam: unremarkable. Neurologic: withdrawal to painful stimuli, moving all extremities.

Laboratory Findings: WBC 18,800/μl, Hct 35.1%. Glucose 115 mg/dl. PT 14.4 sec (control 11.4 sec). ABG (100% O_2 non-rebreathing mask): pH 7.45, pCO_2 32 mmHg, pO_2 105 mmHg, HCO_3^- 22 mEq/L, SaO_2 98%. Chest radiograph (see below): cardiomegaly, infiltrate at the right base.

Hospital Course: The patient experienced convulsions, and he was given intravenous phenytoin and diazepam. He was electively intubated to protect the airway. A nasogastric tube was inserted and gastric lavage was performed using an ice-saline solution.

Question: What is the cause of the patient's high temperature and fever?

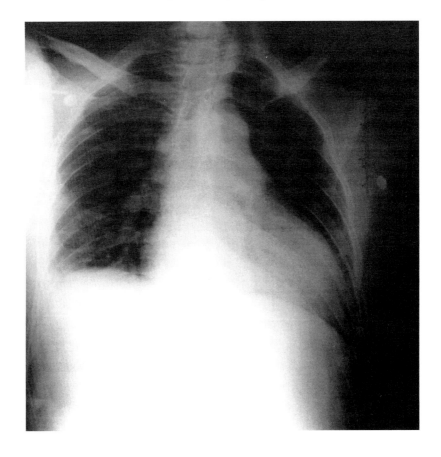

Diagnosis: Heat stroke.

Discussion: Heat stroke is a potentially life-threatening disorder of thermal regulation that occurs mostly in hot, humid weather. It is in this type of weather that the body's two main mechanisms of cooling are impaired. The high heat limits radiant cooling, and the high ambient humidity limits dissipation of heat through evaporation of sweat. These circumstances can be aggravated by factors that generate more heat, such as exercise, although in vulnerable patients such as the elderly no exertion at all is needed to provoke heat stroke.

In 1995, a 5-day heat wave in the city of Chicago was associated with more than 700 deaths, most of which were directly related to heat-associated injury. The ambient temperature during this time period was 93°–104° F, with a heat index as high as 119° F. A case-matched control study of these deaths indicated the following risk factors for heat-related mortality: underlying medical illness resulting in confinement to bed or inability to care for oneself, not leaving one's residence daily, living alone, and living on the top floor of a building. Interestingly, social contacts involving group activities with friends were found to be protective. In a multivariate analysis, being confined to bed and living alone were the strongest predictors of death, and having access to air conditioning and transportation were most strongly protective. Other risk factors for heat stroke identified in previous studies include dehydration and the use of diuretics, as well as obesity, diabetes, and the use of neuroleptic agents.

The clinical findings in heat stroke include lethargy, tachycardia, and hypotension. Laboratory abnormalities include leukocytosis, thrombocytopenia, and an elevated prothrombin time, which may herald the development of disseminated intravascular coagulation. Renal and hepatic dysfunction are also common. Elevations of creatine kinase and the development of rhabdomyolysis may occur, but these complications are typically more common in **exertional** rather than **classic** heat stroke.

Heat stroke is a medical emergency that must be quickly identified and treated. Mortality rises sharply at temperatures > 106° F. The principal objective in treating the patient with heat stroke is reduction of body temperature and its attendant increased oxygen requirement by rapid **lowering of the rectal temperature** to < 102°. All clothing should be removed and general cooling should be initiated. The environment should be cool, ice packs may be applied if available, and the patient can be sprayed with cool water and then fanned to facilitate evaporative cooling. Immersion in ice water is controversial, and iced gastric lavage usually is unnecessary.

Fluid replacement must be performed carefully, especially in patients with heat-related renal failure, to prevent over-hydration and acute pulmonary edema. Hypophosphatemia, hypocalcemia, and hypoglycemia are common, and should be monitored. Establishment of a proper airway, treatment of convulsions, and monitoring for arrhythmias may improve overall outcome in these patients.

The present patient was unusual in that he had no obvious risk factor for heat stroke. He responded well to cooling and awoke and was extubated within a day of admission.

Clinical Pearls

1. Body temperatures > 106° F combined with early elevation of liver enzyme levels strongly suggest the possibility of heat stroke and represent a substantial risk of mortality.

2. Radiation and convection account for about 75% of heat losses at room temperature when an individual is undressed.

3. Risk factors for heat stroke include advanced age and confinement to bed.

4. Rapid cooling usually can be achieved by removing clothing and applying cool water and a fan to speed evaporational heat loss.

REFERENCES

1. Carlson RW, Sakha F. Unraveling the mysteries of heatstroke. Crit Care Med 1996;24:1101.
2. Semenza JC, Rubin CH, Falter KH, et al. Heat-related deaths during the July 1995 heat wave in Chicago. N Engl J Med 1996;335:84–90.
3. Bouchama A. Heatstroke: A new look at an ancient disease. Intensive Care Med 1995;21:623–625.
4. Tan W, Herzlich BC, Funaro R, et al. Rhabdomyolysis and myoglobinuric acute renal failure associated with classic heat stroke. South Med J 1995;88:1065–1068.
5. Costrini A. Emergency treatment of exertional heatstroke and comparison of whole body cooling techniques. Med Sci Sports Exerc 1990;22:15.

PATIENT 55

A 32-year-old woman with difficulty breathing

A 32-year-old woman was brought to the emergency room after being trapped in a fire in her home in which only two of her three children survived. The patient had no significant medical history and was taking no medications.

Physical Examination: Temperature 98.6°; pulse 88; respirations 24 and labored; blood pressure 124/72. General: patient smelled of smoke. HEENT: mild erythema of upper eyelids, singed nose hairs, black debris on lips and tongue. Chest: inspiratory stridor noted. Cardiac: normal. Abdomen: normal. Extremities: burns to both hands. Neurologic: lethargic, but nonfocal.

Laboratory Findings: WBC 11,600/μl, Hct 36.8%. LDH 629 IU/L, CK 522 IU/L. ABG (100% non-rebreathing mask): pH 7.31, pCO_2 52 mmHg, pO_2 101 mmHg, HCO_3^- 26 mEq/L. SaO_2 97%, COHb 13%. Chest radiograph: see below.

Hospital Course: The patient was intubated orally with a 7.5 mm endotracheal tube. There was upper airway edema noted during the intubation.

Question: What is the cause of the patient's respiratory acidosis?

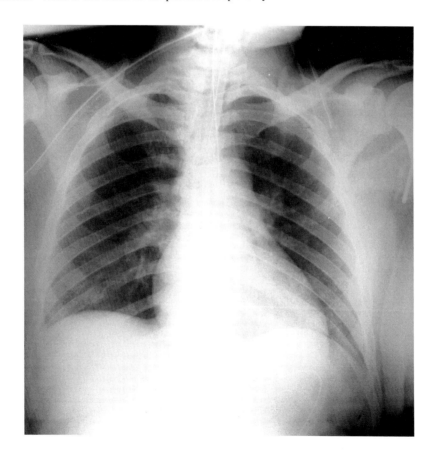

Diagnosis: Upper airway burn injury.

Discussion: Burn injuries and the inhalation of smoke are leading causes of morbidity and mortality in the United States. Respiratory failure is the main cause of death in burn patients, and the predominant factor in the lung damage is smoke inhalation insult.

As noted in a previous case (Patient 26), smoke inhalation injury can result from **three different mechanisms:** a thermal burn to the upper airway, damage to the lungs caused by inhaling the products of combustion, and asphyxiation and neurologic damage caused by carbon monoxide breathing and the formation of carboxyhemoglobin.

Heat inhalation injuries selectively damage the upper airway since breathing in flame and hot gases typically does not result in heat transport down to the lung tissue. The water vapor in the air in the tracheobronchial tree effectively absorbs this heat. Steam inhalation is an exception because it is already superheated water vapor. As a result of the heat injury, tissue edema occurs just as it does with surface burns. However, the site of edema in heat inhalation is the loose mucosa in the supraglottic area, and this damage can progress to complete **airway obstruction** and death. Additionally, due to irritation of inflamed tissue, lethal laryngospasm may occur when the endotracheal tube first touches the laryngeal area.

The only way to *directly* assess thermal injury to the upper airway is by direct visualization, but facial burns and singed eyebrows or nasal hairs are indicators of possible upper airway burn. Another clue is that significant smoke-related injury is more likely to occur in closed spaces. Although clinical evidence of upper airway dysfunction is often delayed in onset, early preventive measures should be initiated to avoid potentially life-threatening problems. Thus, it often is preferable to electively **intubate** patients felt to be at significant risk for upper airway obstruction due to burn injury than to face respiratory arrest later on in an unprotected patient.

Upper airway injury from heat and chemicals in smoke can be detected by direct laryngoscopy. However, the exact degree of injury and risk of worsening edema cannot be accurately predicted by initial findings. In the absence of a critical burn, particularly one that involves the face, the injury often can be treated without intubation. The presence of a deep facial burn leads to massive facial edema, making airway visualization and access extremely difficult, if not impossible. Therefore, early elective intubation is indicated in the presence of deep facial burns.

Routine administration of antibiotics is not recommended in patients with airway burns, as infection usually does not accompany the syndrome, and injudicious use of broad spectrum antibacterials may select out resistant organisms. If extensive mucosal injury is present, however, antibiotics may be warranted. Corticosteroids do not seem to prevent complications of smoke inhalation, but they are indicated in a patient with airflow obstruction not responsive to routine bronchodilators.

The present patient was managed with fluids, antibiotics, prednisone, and aerosolized bronchodilators and was rapidly weaned to extubation 24 hours following admission.

Clinical Pearls

1. Even in the absence of apparent respiratory distress, the patient with facial burns or singed nasal hairs should be carefully evaluated for early airway intervention.

2. Although routine administration of antibiotics and corticosteroids is not indicated in all burn patients, those with extensive mucosal burns and airflow obstruction not responsive to bronchodilators may benefit from these therapies.

3. Pulmonary complications cause or directly contribute to death in 77% of patients with combined inhalation and cutaneous burn injury.

REFERENCES

1. Darling GE, Keresteci MA, Ibanez D, et al. Pulmonary complications in inhalation injuries with associated cutaneous burn. J Trauma 1996;40:83–89.
2. Loick HM, Traber TD, Stothert JC, et al. Smoke inhalation causes a delayed increase in airway blood flow to primarily uninjured lung areas. Intensive Care Med 1995;21:326–333.
3. Demling R, Lalonde C, Youn YK, Picard L. Effect of graded increases in smoke inhalation injury on the early systemic response to a body burn. Crit Care Med 1995;23:171–178.
4. Fitzpatrick JC, Cioffi WG Jr, Cheu HW, Pruitt BA Jr. Predicting ventilation failure in children with inhalation injury. J Pediatr Surg 1994;29:1122–1126.
5. Wittram C, Kenny JB. The admission chest radiograph after acute inhalation injury and burns. Br J Radiol 1994;67:751–754.

PATIENT 56

A 55-year-old woman with shortness of breath and chest pressure

A 55-year-old woman was admitted to the emergency department complaining of severe shortness of breath and mid-sternal chest pressure of eight-hour duration. She had a history of insulin-dependent diabetes mellitus, peripheral vascular disease, and severe coronary artery disease. A recent echocardiogram revealed an ejection fraction of approximately 30% with global hypokinesis. Medications included dipyridamole, regular insulin, captopril, and nitroglycerin.

Physical Examination: Temperature 99°; pulse 68; respirations 20; blood pressure 94/58. Chest: bibasilar inspiratory crackles to the lung apices. Cardiac: jugular venous distention noted, no murmurs or rubs. Abdomen: normal. Extremities: without edema. Neurologic: normal.

Laboratory Findings: WBC 5700/µl, Hct 39%. LDH 509 IU/L, CK 832 IU/L. ABG (non-rebreathing mask): pH 7.43, pCO_2 28 mmHg, pO_2 45 mmHg, HCO_3^- 18 mEq/L, SaO_2 82%. Chest radiograph (see below): perihilar pulmonary vascular congestion. EKG: 1.5 mm ST segment elevation in leads II, III, and aVF.

Hospital Course: The patient was transferred to the CCU, electively intubated, and placed on a Siemens Servo 900C ventilator with the following settings: volume control, V_t 500 ml, f = 16, FiO_2 .90, and PEEP 5 cm H_2O. Arterial blood pressure was maintained with a saline fluid challenge and infusions of dobutamine (20 µg/kg/min) and dopamine (20 µg/kg/min). Pulmonary artery and foley catheters were inserted. CO 2.2 L/min, CI 1.5 L/min/m², PAS/PAD 58/28 mmHg, PCWP 28 mmHg, SvO_2 65%. PEEP was increased incrementally to 20 cm H_2O. Repeat ABG (FiO_2 .90): pH 7.47, pCO_2 34 mmHg, pO_2 90 mmHg, HCO_3^- 20 mEq/L, SaO_2 98%. Hemodynamic indices: blood pressure 115/70, CO 4.4 L/min, CI 3.0 L/min/m², SvO_2 75%.

Questions: What is the most likely diagnosis in this patient? What are the likely mechanisms for the increase in blood pressure, cardiac output, and cardiac index?

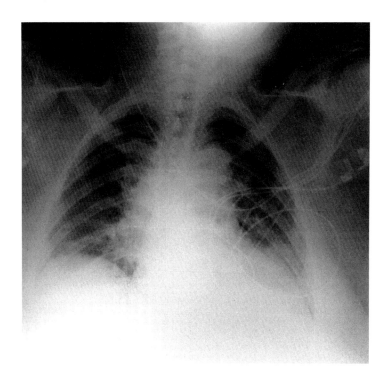

Diagnosis: Acute myocardial infarction with pulmonary edema.

Discussion: Acute myocardial infarction involves death of a portion of the heart muscle due to a deprivation of its blood supply. Pulmonary edema is an increase in pulmonary extravascular water that results when fluid transudation or exudation exceeds the capacity of lymphatic drainage. Pulmonary edema most commonly occurs as a clinical manifestation of left ventricular failure, which is either chronic or, as in the setting of a myocardial infarction, acute.

Pulmonary edema develops in **three stages**. Stage one (interstitial pulmonary edema) is the mildest form of pulmonary edema. There is an increase in interstitial fluid but without passage of edema fluid into the alveoli. While histopathologic examination might reveal cuffs of distended lymphatics, clinical signs are generally absent in stage one, and the diagnosis rests primarily on radiographic findings and associated clinical presentation.

Stage two (crescentic alveolar filling) features increases in extravascular lung water, resulting in fluid passing into some alveolar spaces. Histopathology reveals crescents of fluid in the angles between adjacent alveolar septae. In this stage, alveoli centers remain clear and gas exchange is not severely abnormal.

Stage three (alveolar flooding) represents the most severe form of pulmonary edema. In this stage, alveoli flood when lung fluid clearance mechanisms become overwhelmed. Clinical manifestations include rales and redistribution of pulmonary blood flow on chest roentgenogram. Gas exchange in the pulmonary capillaries is ineffective due to venous admixture or shunt.

The relationship between fluid flow and the balance of pressures is governed by Starling's law of transcapillary exchange and can be best represented by the Starling equation:

$$\dot{Q} = K[Pmv - Ppmv) - \Sigma(\pi mv - \pi pmv)]$$

where $\dot{Q}$ = flow rate of transudated fluid, K = hydraulic conductance, Pmv = hydrostatic pressure in the microvasculature, Ppmv = hydrostatic pressure in the perimicrovascular tissue, Σ = reflection coefficient, πmv = osmotic pressure within microvasculature, and ppmv = osmotic pressure in perimicrovascular tissue. Fluid movement out of the capillary occurs whenever the difference between capillary and interstitial hydrostatic pressure is greater than the difference between capillary and interstitial oncotic pressure.

In an acute myocardial infarction, pulmonary edema may occur as a result of several derangements. In **inferior wall** infarction (which is likely the case with the patient presented here, as the EKG demonstrates ST-segment elevations in leads II, III, and aVF), papillary muscle dysfunction may cause transient mitral valve regurgitation and elevated left atrial pressures leading to pulmonary edema. Such valvular dysfunction often is transient, and patients can generally be managed through this complication. Papillary muscle rupture is more serious, and valve replacement in the setting of an acute myocardial infarction may have to be attempted to save the patient's life. In **anterior wall** infarction, a greater segment of myocardium is at risk, and a large infarct can result in acute left ventricular failure. Pulmonary edema in this setting is associated with substantial mortality. Overall, the occurrence of any degree of pulmonary edema during the course of an acute myocardial infarction is a poor prognostic factor associated with a higher chance of in-hospital death.

The highest priority in pulmonary edema is to **restore arterial pO$_2$**. This is extremely important for ischemic myocardium. Aside from revascularization of the coronary arteries themselves, treatment for the excess lung water includes diuretics and vasodilators (to decrease pre-load). Positive-pressure ventilation reduces ventilation/perfusion mismatching by allowing recruitment of alveolar spaces and also may reduce preload directly by decreasing venous return. Over the past few years, evidence has accumulated that noninvasive ventilation with CPAP or BiPAP also may be an effective way to improve gas exchange in patients with pulmonary edema in the setting of myocardial dysfunction. The essential feature of all positive-pressure ventilation is reduction of left atrial pressure.

The present patient suffered an inferior wall myocardial infarction, complicated by pulmonary edema. She was treated with diuresis, inotropes, mechanical ventilation, and anticoagulation. She improved steadily and was discharged 9 days after admission.

Clinical Pearls

1. The normal lymphatic drainage from human lungs is only about 10 ml per hour; however, lymphatic flow can increase significantly when transudation into the interstitial space increases.

2. The four factors affecting cardiac performance are preload, afterload, heart rate, and contractility.

3. Improvement in gas exchange in pulmonary edema treated with positive-pressure ventilation of any type is due to recruitment of alveolar spaces as well as to reduction in preload associated with positive-pressure breathing.

REFERENCES

1. Fernandez Mondejar E, Vazquez Mata G, Cardenas A, et al. Ventilation with positive end-expiratory pressure reduces extravascular lung water and increases lymphatic flow in hydrostatic pulmonary edema. Crit Care Med 1996;24:1562–1567.
2. Newberry DL 3rd, Noblett KE, Kolhouse L. Noninvasive bilevel positive-pressure ventilation in severe acute pulmonary edema. Am J Emerg Med 1995;13:479–482.
3. Xie SL, Reed RK, Bowen BD. A model of human microvascular exchange. Microvasc Res 1995;49:141–162.
4. Lapinsky SE, Mount DB, Mackey D, et al. Management of acute respiratory failure due to pulmonary edema with nasal positive pressure support. Chest 1994;105:229–231.
5. Brezins M, Benari B, Papo V, et al. Left ventricular function in patients with acute myocardial infarction, acute pulmonary edema, and mechanical ventilation: Relationship to prognosis. Crit Care Med 1993;21:380–385.

PATIENT 57

A 27-year-old woman with kyphoscoliosis and progressive shortness of breath

A 27-year-old woman with severe kyphoscoliosis was brought to the emergency department with progressive shortness of breath for 3 days and abnormal mentation for 1 day. She had been intubated previously for respiratory failure. She had an advance directive which included a "Do Not Intubate" order.

Physical Examination: Temperature 98.6°; pulse 92; respirations 22 and labored; blood pressure 135/76. Chest: clear to auscultation with diminished air entry and distant breath sounds. Cardiac: normal. Abdomen: normal. Extremities: cyanotic. Neurologic: drowsy but easily aroused, otherwise normal. Musculoskeletal: severe lateral scoliosis and anteroposterior curvature of the spine.

Laboratory Findings: WBC 8,000/μl, Hct 57%, platelets 185,000/μl. ABG (room air): pH 7.37, pCO_2 68 mmHg, pO_2 38 mmHg, HCO_3^- 40 mEq/L, SaO_2 71%. Chest radiograph: small lung volumes without infiltrates.

Questions: What explains this patient's respiratory failure? What measures can be taken to reverse it?

Diagnosis: Respiratory failure due to severe kyphoscoliosis.

Discussion: Hypoxia is defined as a reduction of oxygen at the tissue level, whereas hypoxemia refers to a diminution of the oxygen content in the blood. There are essentially four causes of hypoxemia: alveolar hypoventilation, diffusion defect, ventilation/perfusion (V/Q) mismatch, and shunt.

Hypoventilation is caused by inadequate minute volume and is always associated with hypercapnia. It results in alveolar hypoxia by reducing the volume of gas ventilating the alveoli. Consequently, there is insufficient arterial oxygen saturation. Common causes of hypoventilation include depression or injury of the respiratory centers of the brain, interference with the nerves supplying the respiratory muscles, altered mechanics of the lung or chest wall, reduced chest wall mobility, and airway obstruction.

Diffusion defects are caused by diseases in which the alveolar-capillary membrane is altered so that diffusion of all gas molecules is impeded. This causes an increase in the alveolar-arterial oxygen tension difference ([A-a]DO$_2$), resulting in arterial hypoxemia. Possible causes of a reduction in oxygen diffusing capacity include decreased capillary transit time, a reduction in the total area of the alveolar-capillary membrane (such as occurs in emphysema), a reduction in pulmonary capillary blood volume (for example in anemia), pulmonary congestion, and so-called alveolar capillary block, which represents a thickening of the interstitial space seen in situations such as interstitial fibrosis. At rest, diffusion limitation contributes to hypoxemia only when D$_L$CO is severely diminished.

V/Q mismatch also can contribute to hypoxemia and in fact is responsible for the large majority of hypoxemia cases. In the normal lung, at normal lung volumes, most of the gas exchange takes place at the bases where the majority of blood flow and ventilation occurs. Most of the total ventilation and even more of the total blood flow go to the gravity-dependent areas. V/Q imbalance occurs in many pulmonary parenchymal and vascular disorders, including pneumonia, atelectasis, and pulmonary embolism. Typically, hypoxemia due to V/Q imbalance improves somewhat when the patient breathes supplemental oxygen.

Anatomic **right-to-left shunting** can occur in a variety of settings, including Eisenmenger's syndrome. Intrapulmonary shunting can be considered an extreme form of V/Q mismatching, where the V/Q ratio is 0. Arterial hypoxia caused by true right-to-left shunting can be distinguished from that caused by V/Q mismatch because shunt-induced hypoxemia is not relieved by increasing the concentration of inspired oxygen—shunted blood does not participate in gas exchange.

In the present patient, at least two mechanisms accounted for her hypoxemia. Patients with kyphoscoliosis are at a severe mechanical disadvantage because their distorted chest wall architecture causes inefficient muscle contraction and increases the work of breathing. This leads to progressive respiratory muscle fatigue and can result in hypoventilation from respiratory muscle exhaustion. In addition, because of poor chest wall expansion, areas of lung in patients with marked kyphoscoliosis become atelectatic, resulting in V/Q imbalance.

Despite the marked degree of hypoxemia and hypercarbia in this patient, she was not intubated because of her previously stated wish. She was treated instead with noninvasive ventilation and improved over several days. She was discharged and is presently maintained on nasal bilevel positive airway pressure at night.

Clinical Pearls

1. Hypoxemia is caused by hypoventilation, diffusion defect, ventilation-perfusion mismatch, or right-to-left shunt.

2. Hypoxemia caused by hypoventilation, diffusion defect, or ventilation-perfusion mismatch is generally responsive to increases in FiO$_2$; hypoxemia caused by right-to-left shunt is responsive to increases in end-expiratory pressure.

3. Noninvasive ventilation can be used to rest fatigued respiratory muscles in patients with respiratory failure associated with musculoskeletal abnormalities.

REFERENCES

1. Netzer N, Werner P, Korinthenberg R. Nasal BiPAP (bilevel positive airway pressure) respiration with controlled respiratory mode in neuromuscular diseases and severe kyphoscoliosis. Pneumologie 1995;49:161S–164S.
2. Jones DJ, Paul EA, Bell JH, Wedzicha JA. Ambulatory oxygen therapy in stable kyphoscoliosis. Eur Respir J 1995;8:819–823.
3. Grassi V, Tantucci C. Respiratory prognosis in chest wall diseases. Monaldi Arch Chest Dis 1993;48:183–187.
4. Zaccaria S, Zaccaria E, Zanaboni S, et al. Home mechanical ventilation in kyphoscoliosis. Monaldi Arch Chest Dis 1993; 48:161–164.
5. Rochester DF. Respiratory muscles and ventilatory failure: 1993 perspective. Am J Med Sci 1993;305:394–402.

PATIENT 58

A 37-year-old man with weakness of the extremities and arthralgia

A 37-year-old man was brought to the emergency department complaining of weakness and joint pain in his knees, elbows, and ankles. He had been diving to a depth of 114 feet with a bottom-time of 22 minutes when his air source became dysfunctional, and he made an emergency ascent to the surface. His symptoms began approximately 20 minutes after emerging from the water.

Physical Examination: Temperature 98.4°; pulse 104; respirations 26; blood pressure 136/92. Chest: clear. Cardiac: normal. Abdomen: normal. Extremities: without cyanosis. Neurologic: alert although anxious, nonfocal.

Laboratory Findings: SaO$_2$ (room air): 95%. Chest radiograph (see below): without infiltrate.

Hospital Course: An intravenous line was established and normal saline was infused at 150 ml/hr. The patient was given 100% oxygen with a non-rebreathing mask. His symptoms remained unrelieved over the subsequent 2 hours.

Questions: What is the cause of the patient's pain? What further therapy, if any, is indicated?

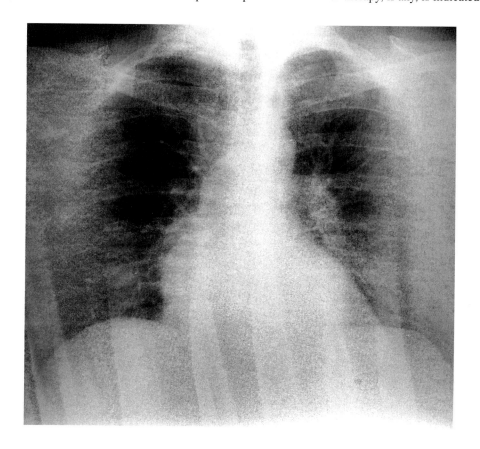

Diagnosis: Decompression sickness (the bends).

Discussion: Decompression sickness is a painful, sometimes fatal syndrome caused by the formation of nitrogen bubbles in the tissues of divers, caisson workers, and aviators who move too rapidly from environments of higher to lower atmospheric pressures. In normal circumstances, nitrogen breathed in air under pressure dissolves in tissue fluids. When ambient pressure is reduced too rapidly, nitrogen comes out of solution faster than it can be circulated to the lungs for expiration. **Gaseous nitrogen** then accumulates in the joint spaces and peripheral circulation, causing pain and impairing tissue oxygenation.

Nitrogen, which accounts for about 80% of the volume of inspired air, is an inert gas that usually dissolves in blood and fat. The inert nature of nitrogen renders this dissolution physiologically meaningless. In contrast to the effects of gases going *into* solution, the effects of gases coming *out* of solution are serious, as is the case in decompression sickness. In slow, controlled ascents, the tissue nitrogen content equilibrates with the alveolar nitrogen content and is eliminated by respiration. In rapid ascents, tissues begin to bubble (off-gas) resulting in mechanical interference with tissue perfusion. Bubbles can form in any tissue but appear to have a predilection for the areas around the joints, spinal cord, brain, and skin. Symptoms commonly consist of arthralgias, paresthesias, and limb weakness.

In addition to tissue involvement, coagulopathies, venous stasis, and hypoxia may be triggered by this process, with potential involvement of other organ systems. Type I decompression sickness can be summarized as mild sickness typically involving only the skin and musculoskeletal systems. Type II decompression sickness is more serious and includes all other potential manifestations of rapid decompression.

Supplemental oxygen should be administered immediately upon recognition of decompression illness, as it washes out blood and tissue nitrogen stores and increases the partial pressure gradient for nitrogen to diffuse from bubbles into tissue or blood. Also, supplemental oxygen hastens bubble shrinkage and ameliorates hypoxia. However, in severe cases of decompression sickness, further therapy will be necessary.

Recompression therapy in a hyperbaric chamber remains the mainstay of treatment for tissue gas. Individuals with gas bubble disease treated early with recompression are more likely to have complete relief of symptoms than those treated after a delay. For the patient who develops serious neurologic symptoms and shows ongoing improvement during the initial recompression or deteriorates during decompression, saturation treatment can be initiated. Saturation treatment consists of a prolonged period of oxygen and air breathing at a specified treatment pressure (often 2 to 3 atmospheres of pressure). Once the patient's condition becomes stabilized, the decompression may be commenced. If a single recompression treatment does not resolve all symptoms, repetitive treatments may produce improvement.

The present patient underwent recompression therapy until he was asymptomatic. He was discharged the next day and received an additional five recompressions at a regional hyperbaric chamber.

Clinical Pearls

1. Duration and depth of descent remain the two most important factors in bubble formation during or after ascent.

2. As a general rule, symptoms that develop within 10 minutes of surfacing are caused by air embolism while symptoms that develop more than 10 minutes after surfacing suggest decompression sickness.

3. Recompression using a hyperbaric chamber reduces the size of nitrogen bubbles, allowing them to be redissolved into the blood stream and eliminated by the lungs.

REFERENCES
1. Burkard ME, Ven Liew HD. Effects of physical properties of the breathing gas on decompression-sickness bubbles. J Appl Physiol 1995;79:1828–1836.
2. Tournebise H, Boucand MH, Landi J, Theobald X. Paraplegia and decompression sickness. Paraplegia 1995;33:636–639.
3. Moon RE, Vann RD, Bennett PB. The physiology of decompression illness. Sci Am 1995;273:70–77.
4. Lee HC, Niu KC, Chen SH, et al. Therapeutic effects of different tables on type II decompression sickness. J Hyperbaric Med 1991;6:11–17.
5. Moon RE. Treatment of gas bubble disease. Probl Respir Care 1991;4:232–252.

PATIENT 59

A 33-year-old man with left-sided chest deformity following an automobile accident

A 33-year-old man was brought to the emergency department by ambulance complaining of dyspnea and left lower chest pain after striking the steering wheel during an automobile accident. The patient was not wearing a seat belt at the time of the accident.

Physical Examination: Temperature 98.6°; pulse 100; respirations 28 with paradoxical chest movement; blood pressure 130/80. General: severe respiratory distress. Chest: left inspiratory crepitus with diminished breath sounds, trachea midline. Cardiac: normal. Abdomen: normal. Extremities: without cyanosis. Neurologic: alert, otherwise normal.

Laboratory Findings: Hct 41.6%. ABG (100% O_2 non-rebreathing mask): pH 7.51, pCO_2 29 mmHg, HCO_3^- 23 mEq/L, pO_2 71 mmHg, SaO_2 96%. Chest radiograph (see below): multiple rib fractures with left-sided infiltrate.

Hospital Course: The patient was electively intubated and mechanical ventilation was initiated with a Siemens Servo 900C with the following settings: SIMV, V_t 800 ml, f = 16, FiO_2 .50, with 6 cm H_2O PEEP.

Question: What is the cause of the patient's respiratory difficulty?

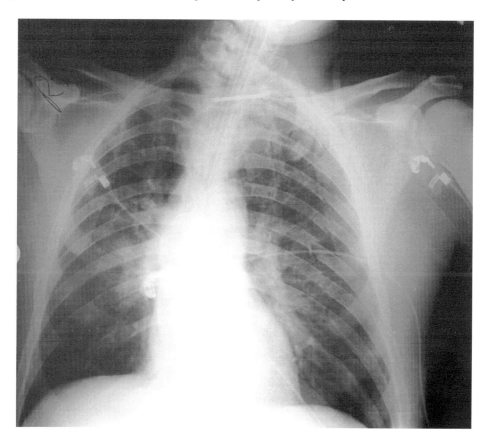

Diagnosis: Flail chest.

Discussion: The term flail chest denotes a condition in which the chest deforms markedly during quiet breathing because of **multiple fractures** of the thoracic cage. Flail chest is produced by segmental rib fractures (i.e., fractures of the same rib in two or more locations) of three or more contiguous ribs, or by combined sternal and rib fractures. These are usually sustained by falls from high places, in automobile accidents, or during cardiac resuscitation. Patients with flail chest frequently have severe associated injuries such as fractures of long bones or vertebrae, head trauma, rupture of the aortic arch or other arteries, and lacerations of the liver or spleen. Primary pulmonary complications associated with the types of trauma that produce flail chest include pulmonary contusion, hemothorax, and pneumothorax.

The physiologic changes that occur with flail chest are interrelated: both ineffective ventilation and increased energy demands of the respiratory muscles are due to the **paradoxical movement** of the flail segment. There also may be hypoxemia secondary to any underlying pulmonary contusion or atelectasis.

The paradoxical movement of the chest wall secondary to loss of the structural integrity of the rib cage reflects the changes in the underlying pleural pressure. Normally, several major forces act on the rib cage during quiet breathing, permitting expansion and relaxation in a uniform fashion. These forces include the passive recoil of the rib cage, the insertional actions of the intercostal muscles and diaphragm, and transthoracic and abdominal pressures. In flail chest, rib fractures uncouple a part of the chest wall from the rib cage, interfering with the actions of the inspiratory muscles. Consequently, during inspiration the collapsing influence of negative intrathoracic pressure is unopposed, so it displaces the uncoupled part of the rib cage inward. During expiration, pleural pressure becomes more positive and moves the flail segment outward. If there is lung contusion or microatelectasis secondary to pain and splinting, the resultant reduction in lung compliance increases the respiratory pressure swings and exacerbates the paradoxical chest wall motion.

Different patterns of chest wall and rib cage distortion can be seen in patients with flail chest. The pattern of paradox may reflect either the location of the rib fractures, or altered recruitment patterns of the respiratory muscles. The paradoxical motion of the chest wall causes the inspiratory muscles to shorten more than usual to produce a given tidal volume. This directly increases the work of breathing by reducing efficiency of respiratory muscles. The combination of increased work and decreased efficiency increases the energy demands and predisposes the muscles to fatigue. Energy supplies to the muscles are further reduced by the presence of hypoxia, predisposing patients with flail chest to even more inspiratory muscle fatigue.

Therapy for flail chest includes pain control and mechanical ventilatory assistance when necessary. The major determinants for the use of mechanical ventilatory support in patients with flail chest include the presence of lung contusion and nonpulmonary complications such as sepsis and arrhythmias. Most patients with flail chest tolerate the problem without significant difficulty if pain is adequately controlled. Mechanical ventilatory support must be used in flail chest injury that is complicated by ventilatory failure or by hypoxic respiratory failure secondary to lung contusion, pneumonia, or acute respiratory distress syndrome. More recently, internal fixation of the ribs as a therapeutic alternative to endotracheal intubation has been advocated. In one study, this approach was associated with a shorter duration of mechanical ventilation and a reduction in the need for tracheostomy.

The present patient was treated with 4 days of mechanical ventilatory support and was rapidly weaned to extubation. He was discharged on day 6 following admission.

Clinical Pearls

1. Flail chest occurs in approximately 20% of patients with blunt chest wall trauma.
2. Lung contusion is a significant component of the flail chest syndrome and is associated with higher rates of complications, morbidity, and mortality.
3. Clinical features suggesting a need for endotracheal intubation include an initial respiratory rate greater than 25, a pulse rate greater than 100, a systolic blood pressure less than 100 mmHg, poor initial arterial blood gas, and the presence of other injuries.

REFERENCES

1. Cappello M, Yuehua C, De Troyer A. Respiratory muscle response to flail chest. Am J Respir Crit Care Med 1996;153:1897–1901.
2. Gregoretti C, Foti G, Beltrame F, et al. Pressure control ventilation and minitracheotomy in treating severe flail chest trauma. Intensive Care Med 1995;21:1054–1056.
3. Ahmed Z, Mohyuddin Z. Management of flail chest injury: Internal fixation versus endotracheal intubation and ventilation. J Thorac Cardiovasc Surg 1995;110:1676–1680.
4. Ciraulo DL, Elliott D, Mitchell KA, Rodriguez A. Flail chest as a marker for significant injuries. J Am Coll Surg 1994;178:466–470.

PATIENT 60

A 53-year-old man with pneumothorax status post esophago-gastrectomy

A 53-year-old man was brought to the post-anesthesia care unit after undergoing an esophago-gastrectomy for esophageal carcinoma. During general anesthesia, it was noted that peak airway pressures were elevated throughout the surgery. Bronchodilators were administered to treat what was thought to be intraoperative bronchospasm. Following reversal of neuromuscular blockade, the patient suddenly developed dyspnea, tachypnea, and right pleuritic chest pain.

Physical Examination: Temperature 99.2°; pulse 108; respirations 36; blood pressure 158/92. Chest: diminished breath sounds on the right side, trachea midline. Cardiac: normal. Abdomen: diminished bowel sounds. Extremities: without cyanosis, clubbing, or edema. Neurologic: normal.

Laboratory Findings: WBC 9400/µl, Hct 44%. ABG (FiO$_2$ .50): pH 7.49, pCO$_2$ 30 mmHg, pO$_2$ 60 mmHg, HCO$_3^-$ 24 mEq/L, SaO$_2$ 92%. Chest radiograph: see below.

Questions: What is the likely cause of the peak airway pressures and diminished breath sounds? What therapy is indicated?

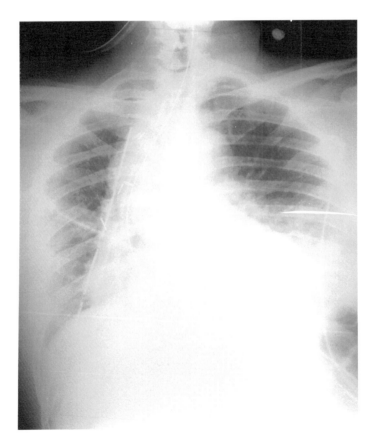

Diagnosis: Pneumothorax.

Discussion: The development of respiratory distress in a patient with an endotracheal tube in place who is receiving mechanical ventilation is a difficult and potentially life-threatening problem. A relatively short list of causes must be reviewed and prompt action taken before significant hypoxemia occurs.

When respiratory distress occurs along with high peak airway pressures, as in this case, the possibilities include bronchospasm and airflow limitation, a mucus plug in the endotracheal tube, slippage of the tube into the right main bronchus, a kink in the endotracheal tube, blockage of the tube by a lightly anesthetized and agitated patient who is struggling and biting, and the development of a pneumothorax. These problems can be differentiated by the physical examination and a chest radiograph. Wheezing is heard only in the case of bronchospasm. A mucus plug may cause extremely high airway pressures, and the patient can be difficult to ventilate even with manual bagging, but no wheezing is heard. Biting or kinking of the endotracheal tube should be fairly obvious. Both a pneumothorax and a right main bronchus intubation are associated with **unilateral diminished breath** sounds, but these two can be easily distinguished on a **chest radiograph**. It is important to remember that a pneumothorax in a supine patient may be manifest solely as a hyperlucency over the mediastinum or at the costophrenic angle (the deep sulcus sign).

Once a diagnosis of pneumothorax has been made in an intubated patient undergoing mechanical ventilation, a **tube thoracostomy** should be performed as soon as possible, as the pneumothorax is under positive pressure and tension may occur. Expectant management of a pneumothorax without a chest tube in a mechanically ventilated patient is almost never indicated. If tension is present (as evidenced by severe respiratory distress, hypotension, and a shift of the trachea away from the side of diminished breath sounds), immediate placement of a small catheter into the second intercostal space in the midclavicular line is advisable. The catheter should be attached to intravenous tubing and the free end of the tubing should be placed in a cup of water to create a water seal. If there is no tension, a standard chest tube can be inserted.

The site of insertion for chest tube placement depends on the substance being removed from the pleural space. The relatively wide, avascular second intercostal space in the midclavicular line is the generally recommended insertion site for a pneumothorax, because air rises to the anterior region of the pleural space in the supine patient. The anterior axillary line at the sixth intercostal space with anterior tube positioning is also appropriate.

When a chest tube is inserted, a **drainage system** should be preselected for connection immediately following the procedure. A one-bottle, water-seal drainage provides no suction but permits removal of air from the pleural space. The chest tube is connected via rubber tubing to a long underwater-seal tube in a transparent water-seal drainage bottle. Another short tube in the bottle acts as an air vent. The underwater-seal tube is positioned 2–3 cm below the surface of the water. When positive pressure in the pleural space exceeds 2 cm H_2O, air or fluid is expelled into the bottle, and air escapes through the air vent.

A two-bottle system is needed for fluid drainage. In the two-bottle system, the first bottle is the trap or drainage bottle and the second bottle acts as the water seal. The drainage bottle facilitates the measurement and observation of chest fluid drainage. It also obviates the need for recurrent manipulation of the water-seal tube, which only needs to be kept 2–3 cm below the surface of the water. Clamping the chest tube should never be done in a ventilated patient, as it is only when the tube is clamped that a tension pneumothorax can occur with a chest tube in place.

A third bottle can be added when continuous suction is needed to manage a persistent air leak and achieve complete lung reexpansion. This suction control bottle adjusts the negative pressure generated by the system. In most hospitals, preconstructed units that have replaced the three-bottle system are available.

The present patient's pneumothorax resolved with the benefit of a chest tube connected to underwater seal with –20 cm H_2O. The lung re-expanded and the chest tube was removed on day 3 following insertion.

Clinical Pearls

1. The differential diagnosis of respiratory distress and high peak airway pressures in a mechanically ventilated patient includes bronchospasm, a mechanical obstruction of the tube (by a mucus plug, for example), a right main bronchus intubation or migration of the tube, kinking or biting of the tube, and pneumothorax.

2. A physical examination and chest radiograph usually allow discrimination of the various causes of respiratory distress in this setting.

3. To relieve a pneumothorax, a chest tube is placed in the second intercostal space in the midclavicular line or the anterior axillary line of the sixth intercostal space. The tube should never be clamped in a ventilated patient because of the risk of tension pneumothorax.

REFERENCES

1. Curtin JJ, Goodman LR, Quebbeman EJ, Haasler GB. Complications after emergency tube thoracostomy: Assessment with CT. Radiology 1996;198:19.
2. Quigley RL. Thoracentesis and chest tube drainage. Crit Care Clin 1995;11:111–126.
3. Kinney MR, Kirchhoff KT, Puntillo KA. Chest tube removal practices in critical care units in the United States. Am J Crit Care 1995;4:419–424.
4. McConaghy PM, Kennedy N. Tension pneumothorax due to intrapulmonary placement of intercostal chest drain. Anaesth Intensive Care 1995;23:496–498.
5. Peek GJ, Firmin RK, Arsiwala S. Chest tube insertion in the ventilated patient. Injury 1995;26:425–426.

PATIENT 61

An 83-year-old woman with pulmonary edema and agitation

The respiratory therapist in the coronary care unit was called to evaluate an 83-year-old woman who was receiving mechanical ventilation for pulmonary edema when she suddenly became agitated, short of breath, and appeared to be fighting the ventilator. Medications included furosemide, captopril, and cholestyramine.

Physical Examination: Temperature 98.7°; pulse 110; respirations 38; blood pressure 150/94. General: diaphoretic. Chest: intercostal retractions and decreased thoracic excursion with mechanical breaths. Cardiac: tachycardic. Abdomen: soft, with bowel sounds. Extremities: without cyanosis or edema. Neurologic: extremely agitated.

Laboratory Findings: Na^+ 131 mEq/L, K^+ 3.7 mEq/L, Cl^- 99 mEq/L. ABG (FiO_2 .40): pH 7.56, pCO_2 26 mm Hg, PO_2 61 mmHg, HCO_3^- 37 mEq/L, SaO_2 94%. Chest radiograph (see below): pulmonary vascular congestion. EKG: sinus tachycardia without ST-T wave abnormalities.

Question: How should the patient's agitation be evaluated and treated?

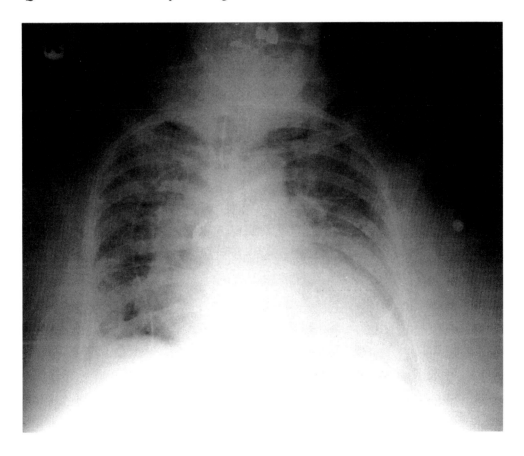

Diagnosis: Ventilation malfunction due to kinking of the ventilator tubing.

Discussion: "Fighting the ventilator" is best described as the presence of agitation and respiratory distress in ventilator-supported patients. Since anxiety is common at the time of intubation in many patients, some degree of fighting is to be expected initially. Accordingly, patients about to be intubated usually receive premedication to facilitate intubation. However, the development of "fighting" in a previously calm patient suggests the likelihood of a new and potentially serious complication. It can be difficult to diagnose the cause of agitation in a mechanically ventilated patient; therefore, patient- and ventilator-related possibilities must be carefully examined.

There are many **patient-related causes** of discomfort on the ventilator, including artificial airway problems, secretions, barotrauma, bronchospasm, pulmonary edema, pulmonary embolism, agitation, and dynamic hyperinflation. **Ventilator-related causes** typically include system leaks, circuit malfunctions, inadequate FiO_2, and inadequate ventilator support. Additionally, patient-ventilator asynchrony may contribute to acute respiratory distress.

Sudden respiratory dysfunction usually results in the development of dyspnea leading to anxiety or agitation, and arterial oxygenation should be assessed immediately in any patient who develops sudden respiratory distress while receiving mechanical ventilation. Tachypnea, diaphoresis, nasal flaring, accessory muscle usage, tachycardia, arrhythmias, and hypotension are several physical signs of respiratory distress. Regardless of the cause of acute respiratory distress in a ventilator-supported patient, the mainstay in management is ensuring the **delivery of adequate ventilation**.

Any mechanically supported patient who becomes suddenly agitated and fights the ventilator should be removed from the machine and provided with a manual resuscitator with 100% supplemental oxygen. If the symptoms are alleviated by this procedure, then it is likely that the ventilator was the cause of the distress. Troubleshooting a ventilator-related cause can usually be accomplished at the bedside while the patient is supported manually. Ventilator problems can include water in the tubing, disconnection of the tubing resulting in a failure of ventilation, or, on rare occasions, failure to provide the indicated amount of inspired oxygen. If the patient remains symptomatic after disconnection from the ventilator, then it is likely that the cause of the distress lies with the patient. A rapid physical examination should be performed and the patency of the airway assessed. If the patient is in extremis, treat the most likely causes until stabilization occurs or a specific diagnosis is achieved.

Patient-ventilator **dissynchrony** occurs when the ventilator settings are not comfortable for the patient, and the patient senses excess work of breathing. This can result from improperly set parameters, such as choosing an uncomfortable ventilatory mode (for example, intermittent mandatory ventilation is likely to be uncomfortable for many patients if pressure support is not added), choosing an uncomfortable waveform, allowing the development of auto-PEEP by not permitting proper expiratory time, or setting the trigger for an assisted breath at an uncomfortably high level. All of these parameters and more should be evaluated in an uncomfortable patient.

The present patient developed agitation and respiratory distress following the kinking of the inspiratory limb of the ventilator circuit by inadvertent positioning of the bedrail. This untoward event was heralded by the sounding of the high pressure limit, low tidal volume, and low minute volume alarms from the ventilator. The situation was corrected and the patient-ventilator synchrony was restored.

Clinical Pearls

1. The persistence of respiratory distress upon disconnecting the patient from the ventilator indicates that the underlying problem is ventilator-based.

2. The cardinal principle of management of sudden respiratory distress is to ensure delivery of adequate ventilation to the patient.

3. Ventilator-supported patients also may develop agitation as a result of pain, anxiety, delirium.

REFERENCES

1. Jubran A, Van de Graaff WB, Tobin MJ. Variability of patient-ventilator interaction with pressure support ventilation in patients with chronic obstructive pulmonary disease. Am J Respir Crit Care Med 1995;152:129–136.
2. Manning HL, Molinary EJ, Leiter JC. Effect of inspiratory flow rate on respiratory sensation and pattern of breathing. Am J Respir Crit Care Med 1995;151:751–757.
3. Marcy TW, Marini JJ. Respiratory distress in the ventilated patient. Clin Chest Med 1994;15:55–73.
4. Manzano JL, Lubillo S, Henriquez D. Verbal communication of ventilator-dependent patients. Crit Care Med 1993;21:512–517.
5. Tobin MJ. What should the clinician do when a patient "fights the ventilator"? Respir Care 1991:36:395–406.

PATIENT 62

An 18-year-old man with no neurologic function 7 days after a gun-shot wound to the cervical spine

An 18-year-old man with a gun-shot wound to the cervical spine was admitted to the emergency department. Following stabilization and surgical removal of a 9-mm bullet, he was transferred to the surgical intensive care unit where he remained ventilator dependent. He had an unremarkable medical history.

Physical Examination: Temperature 99.1°; pulse 76; respirations 12, assisted; blood pressure 116/62. Chest: clear. Cardiac: normal. Neck: posterior pull entry and exit wound. Neurologic: quadriplegia at C4 level.

Laboratory Findings: WBC 8700/μl, Hct 42%. ABG (FiO_2 .30): pH 7.39, pCO_2 39 mmHg, pO_2 106 mmHg, HCO_3^- 25 mEq/L. SaO_2 98%. Chest radiograph: see below.

Question: Should the patient undergo tracheostomy for long-term ventilatory support?

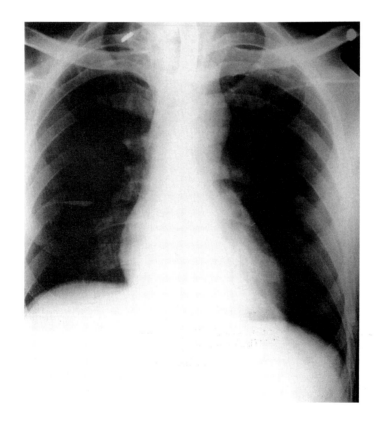

Answer: Tracheostomy should be performed at the first opportunity after the patient stabilizes.

Discussion: The major general indications for tracheostomy include relief of upper airway obstruction, facilitation of pulmonary toilet, and control of the airway in patients requiring prolonged mechanical ventilatory support. In addition, in patients requiring long-term ventilatory support, tracheostomy usually is a more comfortable approach to the airway than translaryngeal intubation.

Tracheostomy may be the initial approach to control of the airway in patients with respiratory emergencies caused by **upper airway obstruction**. Patients with a variety of neoplastic, infectious, or functional disorders that compromise ventilation may require tracheostomy urgently, though the placement of emergency tracheostomy tubes differs somewhat from electively created stomas.

Tracheostomy is also used in the patient with **poor control of airway secretions**. Patients experiencing glottic dysfunction due to trauma or cerebrovascular disease may require tracheostomy to prevent aspiration of particulates and also to facilitate their removal by frequent airway suctioning. Suctioning of the lower respiratory tract is more efficiently accomplished through a tracheostomy tube than through most endotracheal tubes.

In the medical setting, the most common indication for tracheostomy is **prolonged mechanical ventilatory support**. Patients with neuromuscular disorders, chronic obstructive lung disease, lung injury, multi-organ system failure, and pneumonia who become ventilator dependent are often converted from translaryngeal intubation to tracheostomy to facilitate care and improve comfort.

The question of the timing of tracheostomy for the intubated patient traditionally is based on an assessment of the advantages and disadvantages of each route of cannulation. Assessments involve evaluation of the risks and complications of tracheostomy compared with the risks and complications of prolonged intubation. The complications associated with tracheostomy include ulceration, bleeding, tracheoesophageal fistula, tracheal stenosis, the potentially life-threatening tracheo-innominate fistula, infection, and mortality from the procedure itself (related mostly to the small risk of general anesthesia). The complications associated with prolonged intubation include ulceration of the vocal cords, posterior commissure syndromes, tracheomalacia, and tracheal stenosis. In addition, patient discomfort is greater with an endotracheal tube in place, and speaking and eating are impossible. Tracheostomy allows greater comfort and the ability to speak or eat if not connected to the ventilator. Moreover, many physicians and respiratory therapists feel that it is easier to wean patients from mechanical ventilation if a tracheostomy tube rather than an endotracheal tube is in place. This may be because of better control of secretions and greater patient comfort with tracheostomy. Currently, however, no data clearly indicate that translaryngeal intubation is unsafe beyond any certain period of time, nor that tracheostomy is riskier than translaryngeal intubation.

In the absence of rigid guidelines, the decision-making process should be flexible and must always be individualized to the specific patient. The aforementioned assessment permits an anticipatory approach based on the timing of the procedure. Tracheostomy should be considered after a patient with acute respiratory failure undergoes a period of stabilization, generally no longer than 7 days. At that time, the duration of anticipated intubation should be estimated. Patients who appear likely to undergo successful extubation within the following 7 days are maintained with a translaryngeal tube until weaning and extubation are accomplished. Patients with severe conditions that forecast continued requirements for intubation for periods in excess of an additional 2 weeks should be considered for early tracheostomy. If the duration of mechanical ventilation cannot be anticipated after the 7-day stabilization period of intubation, then the patient should be reevaluated on a daily basis.

As the present patient requires life-long ventilatory support due to his spinal cord injury, a decision to perform a tracheostomy was made as soon as the patient was otherwise medically stable.

Clinical Pearls

1. The decision to perform a tracheostomy is dependent on a patient's individual clinical condition and the risks and benefits associated with tracheostomy versus translaryngeal intubation.

2. A tracheostomy places a patent airway below the critical level of the larynx that is predisposed to complications from a translaryngeal endotracheal tube.

3. Translaryngeal endotracheal intubation exceeding 7 days is considered prolonged and thus encourages an anticipatory approach to determining future airway management requirements.

REFERENCES

1. Richard I, Giraud M, Perrouin-Verbe B, et al. Laryngotracheal stenosis after intubation or tracheostomy in patients with neurological disease. Arch Phys Med Rehabil 1996;77:493–496.
2. Friedman Y, Fildes J, Mizock B, et al. Comparison of percutaneous and surgical tracheostomies. Chest 1996;110:480–485.
3. Massard G, Rouge C, Dabbagh A, et al. Tracheobronchial lacerations after intubation and tracheostomy. Ann Thorac Surg 1996;61(5):1483–1487.
4. Neri M, Donner CF, Grandi M, Robert D. Timing of tracheostomy in neuromuscular patients with chronic respiratory failure. Monaldi Arch Chest Dis 1995;50:220–222.
5. Heffner JE. Timing of tracheostomy in mechanically ventilated patients. Am Rev Respir Dis 1993;147:768–771.

PATIENT 63

A 48-year-old man with refractory hypoxemia and pneumonia

A 48-year-old obese man was admitted to the hospital with a left lower lobe pneumonia and refractory hypoxemia. He was treated with intravenous ciprofloxacin and ceftazidime. Twenty-four hours after admission he became severely dyspneic. His medical history included hypertension, hypercholesterolemia, non–insulin-dependent diabetes mellitus, and peripheral vascular disease.

Physical Examination: Temperature 101.7°; pulse 90; respirations 26; blood pressure 136/72. Chest: decreased breath sounds over the left lower lobe with rhonchi throughout. Cardiac: regular rhythm without rubs. Abdomen: nontender, without organomegaly. Extremities: no cyanosis, clubbing, or edema. Neurologic: nonfocal.

Laboratory Findings: WBC 13,700/μl, Hct 41%, platelets 330,000/μl. K^+ 3.4 mEq/L, glucose 167 mg/dl. ABG (FiO_2 .75): pH 7.37, pCO_2 26 mmHg, pO_2 55 mmHg, HCO_3^- 18 mEq/L, SaO_2 89%. Sputum Gram stain: gram-negative rods. Chest radiograph (see below): left-sided infiltrate.

Hospital Course: The patient was intubated and placed on a Siemens Servo 900C ventilator with the following settings: PCV 38 cm H_2O, f = 26, FiO_2 1.0, and PEEP of 10 cm H_2O. Repeat ABG: pH 7.34, pCO_2 22 mmHg, pO_2 58 mmHg, HCO_3^- 19 mEq/L, SaO_2 90%. On repeat chest radiograph, no improvement was noted.

Question: What ventilatory strategies are available for a patient with severe hypoxemia and unilateral lung disease?

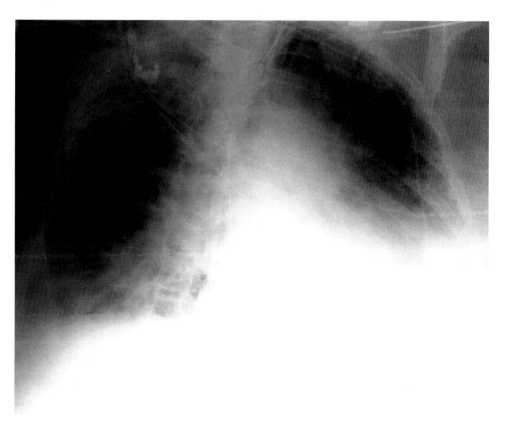

Diagnosis: Severe lobar pneumonia.

Discussion: The pathophysiology of severe hypoxemia in the setting of asymmetric lung disease (for example, acute lobar pneumonia, as in the present patient) is probably largely explained by extreme **ventilation/perfusion (V/Q) mismatching** and/or shunt. When the pneumonia develops rapidly and fills the alveolar spaces of an entire lobe with pus, inflammatory cells, and fluid, the pulmonary blood flow to the region is not shifted away immediately, resulting in severe abnormalities of gas exchange. Thus, strategies to improve gas exchange attempt to restore some balance of ventilation and perfusion.

One of the simplest approaches is to position the patient in the lateral recumbent position, with the unaffected side down on the bed, so that blood flow to the "good" side improves, aided by gravity. This approach has been shown to improve gas exchange dramatically in some patients. However, the technique runs the risk of spilling secretions to the unaffected lung, or of dislodging the endotracheal tube as the patient is turned.

A second strategy is **independent lung ventilation (ILV)**. ILV has changed the approach to the ventilatory support of patients with unilateral lung disease because it allows differential delivery of gas in a manner appropriate to the disease state of the affected lung and to the responsiveness of the unaffected, contralateral lung. Conditions for which ILV commonly is used include correction of severe life-threatening hypoxia due to V/Q mismatching in the setting of unilateral lung disease, selective airway protection (such as in a case of massive hemoptysis), management of bronchopleural fistulae, and single lung transplantation.

Prior to implementing ILV, a double-lumen endobronchial tube (DLEB) must be inserted. There are a number of DLEB tubes available, but because of the short length of the right mainstem bronchus before the origin of the right upper-lobe interval, left-sided endobronchial intubation is more practical and safer than right-sided intubation. Following tube placement and after the tracheal section of the tube is occluded and the bronchial port ventilated, auscultation should be performed. Chest radiography is necessary to further confirm tube position; bronchoscopy is optional.

A variety of techniques for ILV are available. **Synchronous** ILV consists of synchronized initiation of inspiration into each lung. The lungs must have the same ventilatory rate but may have different tidal volumes, PEEP, and inspiratory flow rates. Typically, two ventilators are linked to cycle synchronously. A single ventilator may be used if it is connected to a twin circuit with devices that create different flows into each circuit, or if it is connected to two circuits, each with a separate PEEP value or other PEEP-generating device.

Asynchronous ILV consists of completely independent ventilatory techniques applied to each lung and requires two separate mechanical ventilators. This technique permits delivery of different ventilatory rates, tidal volumes, inspiratory flow rates, and PEEP to each lung.

The present patient had lobar consolidation of his left lower lobe. He was reintubated using a DLEB tube and asynchronous ILV was initiated with the following settings:

Left lung—PCV 38 cm H_2O, f = 30, FiO_2 1.0, PEEP 10 cm H_2O, C_L 17 cc/cm H_2O

Right lung—PCV 26 cm H_2O, f = 22, FiO_2 1.0, PEEP 6 cm H_2O, C_L 31 cc/cm H_2O.

Repeat ABG: pH 7.38, pCO_2 30 mmHg, pO_2 81, HCO_3^- 20 mEq/L, SaO_2 95%. The patient's pneumonia responded to antibiotic therapy and he was successfully weaned and extubated on day 8 following intubation.

Clinical Pearls

1. Patients with severe, acute, unilateral lung disease may develop profound hypoxemia due to extensive ventilation/perfusion mismatching and shunt.

2. Independent lung ventilation is justified when conventional ventilatory support fails in any patient with acute asymmetrical lung injury.

3. Occlusion of the right upper lobe bronchus is known to occur in 89% of patients with a right-sided, double-lumen endobronchial tube; therefore, left-sided tubes are recommended.

REFERENCES

1. Charan NB, Carvalho CG, Hawk P, et al. Independent lung ventilation with a single ventilator using a variable resistance valve. Chest 1995;107:256–260.
2. Badesch DB, Zamora MR, Jones S, et al. Independent ventilation and ECMO for severe unilateral pulmonary edema after SLT for primary pulmonary hypertension. Chest 1995;107:1766–1770.
3. Lohse AW, Klein O, Hermann E, et al. Pneumatoceles and pneumothoraces complicating staphylococcal pneumonia: Treatment by synchronous independent lung ventilation. Thorax 1993;48:578–580.
4. Dreyfuss D, Djedaini K, Lanore JJ, et al. A comparative study of the effects of almitrine bismesylate and lateral position during unilateral bacterial pneumonia with severe hypoxemia. Am Rev Respir Dis 1992;146:295–299.
5. Alberti A, Valenti S, Gallo F. Differential lung ventilation with a double-lumen tracheostomy tube in unilateral refractory atelectasis. Intens Care Med 1992;18:479–484.

PATIENT 64

A 29-year-old woman with cystic fibrosis, productive cough, and fever

A 29-year-old woman presented to her physician's office with productive cough and fever of 2-day duration. Since shortly after birth, she has been followed routinely in the cystic fibrosis clinic. Medications included ibuprofen, terfenadine, DNase, pancrelipase, flunisolide, salmeterol and albuterol inhalers, and vitamins A, D, E, and K. Past sputum cultures were positive for *Pseudomonas cepacia* and *Staphylococcus aureus*.

Physical Examination: Temperature 100°; pulse 88; respirations 26; blood pressure 128/90. Chest: rhonchi throughout. Cardiac: tachycardic. Abdomen: without organomegaly. Extremities: no cyanosis, clubbing, or edema. Neurologic: normal.

Laboratory Findings: SpO$_2$ (room air): 92%. PFT: FVC 2.22 L (65% predicted), post bronchodilator FVC 2.29 L; FEV$_1$ 1.65 L (55% predicted), post bronchodilator FEV$_1$ 1.75 L; DLCO 15.4 ml/min/mmHg (75% predicted). Chest radiograph: see below.

Question: What therapeutic approaches are available for this exacerbation of the patient's cystic fibrosis?

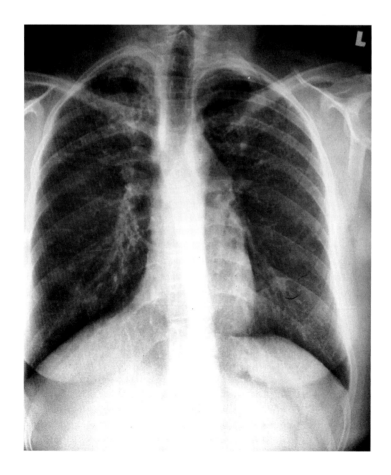

Answer: Cystic fibrosis (CF) is a genetic disorder that presents as a multisystem disease, though the clinical syndrome is dominated by chronic respiratory illness and infection. Typically, the first signs and symptoms occur in childhood, but nearly 3% of patients are diagnosed as adults. The disease is characterized by **chronic airway infection** that ultimately leads to bronchiectasis, as well as exocrine pancreatic insufficiency, abnormal sweat gland function, and urogenital dysfunction.

CF is inherited as an autosomal recessive disease and its prevalence varies with the ethnic origin of a population. It is detected in 1 in 2500 live births of the Caucasian population of North America and northern Europe, 1 in 17,000 live births of African-Americans, and 1 in 90,000 live births of the Asian population of Hawaii. CF is now known to arise as a result of mutations in a gene called the cystic fibrosis transmembrane conductance regulator (CFTR). CFTR functions as a chloride channel, and the most common mutation (called ΔF508) causing the disease results in a single amino acid change at position 508 in the CFTR protein. The carrier frequency of the recessive trait is estimated to be 1 in 30 among Caucasians.

The central hypothesis of CF airways pathophysiology is that the abnormal sodium and chloride transport rates produce secretions that are dehydrated and poorly cleared. The unique predisposition of CF airways to chronic infection by *Staphylococcus aureus* and *Pseudomonas cepacia* indicates that other as yet undefined abnormalities in airway surface liquids also may contribute to the failure of lung defenses.

The diagnosis of CF rests on a combination of clinical criteria and analyses of sweat chloride values. The values for the sodium and chloride concentration in sweat vary with age, but typically in adults a chloride concentration of greater than 70 mEq/L discriminates between CF patients and patients with other lung disease.

Upper respiratory tract disease is almost universal in CF patients. Chronic sinusitis is common in childhood and leads to nasal obstruction and rhinorrhea. The occurrence of nasal polyps approaches 20% and often requires surgery. In the lower respiratory tract, the first symptom of CF is cough. With time, the cough becomes continuous and produces viscous, purulent, and often greenish sputum. Inevitably, periods of clinical stability are interrupted by exacerbations which are defined by increased cough, weight loss, increased sputum volume, and decrements in pulmonary function. These exacerbations typically are treated with intravenous antibiotics with recovery of most lung function during the early course of the disease. Over the course of years, the exacerbations become more frequent with incomplete recovery of lost lung function, ultimately leading to respiratory failure.

The presence of an increased residual volume/total lung capacity ratio in children suggests that small airways disease is the first functional lung abnormality detected in CF. As the disease progresses, both reversible and irreversible changes in FVC and FEV_1 are observed. The reversible component reflects accumulation of intraluminal secretions and/or airway reactivity while the irreversible component reflects chronic destruction of the airway wall and bronchiectasis.

The major objectives of therapy for CF are to promote clearance of secretions and control infection in the lung, provide adequate nutrition, and prevent intestinal obstruction. Techniques for clearing pulmonary secretions include a combination of breathing exercises and chest percussion. Pharmacologically, acetylcysteine has not been shown to have clinically significant effects on mucus clearance or lung function. However, agents that degrade the high concentrations of DNA in CF sputum, such as human recombinant DNAse, appear to be effective in decreasing sputum viscosity and increasing airflow during short-term administration. The long-term benefit of DNAse therapy has not been demonstrated.

Antibiotics are the principal agents available for treating lung infection, and their use should be guided by sputum culture results. Early intervention with antibiotics is useful, and long courses of treatment are the rule. Because of the increased total-body clearance and volume of distribution of antibiotics in CF patients, the required doses are higher for CF patients than for non-CF patients with similar chest infections.

Maintenance of adequate nutrition is critical for the health of the CF patient. Over 90% of CF patients benefit from pancreatic enzyme replacement. The dose of enzymes should be adjusted on the basis of weight gain, abdominal symptomatology, and character of stools. Replacement of fat soluble vitamins (A, D, E, and K) is also required.

In the past several years, double lung transplantation has been successfully used in the treatment of CF. Both lungs must be replaced so that all infected tissue is removed. Ultimately, gene therapy may be the treatment of choice.

The present patient was treated at home parenterally using a third generation cephalosporin (ceftazidime) in conjunction with an aminoglycoside (tobramycin).

Clinical Pearls

1. The diagnosis of cystic fibrosis rests on the demonstration of an elevated sweat chloride concentration in association with either chronic pulmonary disease or pancreatic insufficiency.

2. Over 95% of cystic fibrosis patients die of complications resulting from lung infection.

3. Therapy with rhDNAse improves pulmonary function in the short term, though long-term benefits of this approach have not been demonstrated.

REFERENCES

1. Balfour-Lynn IM, Dinwiddie R. Role of corticosteroids in cystic fibrosis lung disease. J Royal Soc Med 1996;89(Suppl 27):8–13.
2. MacDonald A. Nutritional management of cystic fibrosis. Arch Dis Child 1996;74:81–87.
3. Ramsey BW. Management of pulmonary disease in patients with cystic fibrosis. N Engl J Med 1996;335:179–188.
4. Kotloff RM, Zuckerman JB. Lung transplantation for cystic fibrosis: Special considerations. Chest 1996;109:787–798.
5. Delaney SJ, Wainwright BJ. New pharmaceutical approaches to the treatment of cystic fibrosis. Nat Med 1996;2:392–393.
6. Fuchs HJ, Borowitz DH, Christiansen EM, et al. Effect of aerosolized recombinant human DNase on exacerbations of respiratory symptoms and on pulmonary function in patients with cystic fibrosis. N Engl J Med 1994;331:637–642.

PATIENT 65

A 3-year-old boy with cystic fibrosis, dyspnea, and wheezing

A 3-year-old boy was brought to his pediatrician for increased dyspnea and wheezing of 2-day duration. Medical history included cystic fibrosis diagnosed at 3 months, pulmonic stenosis, and recurrent otitis media. Medications included albuterol, beclomethasone, cromolyn sodium, pancreplipase, vitamins A, D, E, and K, and trimethoprim/sulfamethoxazole.

Physical Examination: Temperature 99.4°; pulse 116, respirations 34; blood pressure 114/76. Chest: bilateral mid-to-end expiratory wheezing with mild substernal retractions, rhonchi throughout. Cardiac: regular rhythm, systolic murmur. Abdomen: scaphoid, without organomegaly. Extremities: no cyanosis, clubbing, or edema. Neurologic: normal.

Laboratory Findings: WBC 9100/μl, Hct 29.9%, Cr 0.2 mg/dl. SpO$_2$ (room air): 91%. Chest radiograph (see below): revealed basilar microatelectasis.

Question: What is the best approach to the treatment of exacerbations of cystic fibrosis?

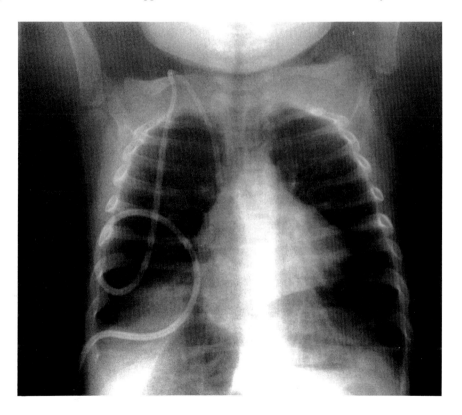

Answer/Discussion: The median age of patients with cystic fibrosis (CF) in the United States is 13 years with a median survival of 29.6 years for men and 27.3 years for women. These survival times represent a substantial improvement; patients with CF once rarely lived beyond their teenage years, but now more and more survive to adulthood. The major improvements in survival are attributable mostly to improved nutritional status provided by digestive supplements, early and aggressive treatment of pulmonary infections, and recognition of and vigorous therapy for the other pulmonary complications of CF, including reactive airway dysfunction, pnuemothorax, and hemoptysis.

Removal of purulent secretions from the lungs of patients with CF has long been a staple of treatment. Pulmonary function test results improve with treatment of an exacerbation with or without antibiotics, illustrating the importance of **pulmonary toilet**. Postural drainage, accompanied by percussion, deep breathing exercises, directed cough, forced expiration technique, and exercise have all been used in clinical practice. A new hand-held instrument, called a flutter device, recently has been introduced to complement these therapies. Exhalation through the device resulting in oscillation of airflow and vibration of airways may improve patient compliance as well as clearance of mucus. Adult patients may choose to substitute programs of exercise for conventional chest physiotherapy. Exercise programs improve maximal oxygen consumption, exercise tolerance, and psychological well-being while decreasing the degree of limitation in activities of daily living.

Oxygen therapy is indicated in patients with CF and exercise-related or resting hypoxemia, or cor pulmonale. Supplemental oxygen alleviates dyspnea associated with exercise-induced arterial desaturation and improves the patient's sense of well-being. Generally, a greater degree of hypoxemia is associated with a worsening of pulmonary hypertension and right-sided heart strain. It has been demonstrated that pulmonary hypertension related to CF can be reduced with oxygen therapy and that the development of cor pulmonale may be prevented through the early use of oxygen.

Oxygen therapy should begin when the patient has nocturnal oxygen desaturation, which may occur even in patients with mild lung disease. Continuous oxygen therapy may become necessary when daytime oxygen saturations begin to fall below 90%, although acceptance of oxygen during the day is sometimes poor. Transtracheal oxygen delivery techniques are more acceptable cosmetically and may become the preferred mode of therapy for younger, more active patients.

Airway hyperreactivity is a common finding in patients afflicted with CF. There is a high rate of within-subject variability in spirometric testing at different times in the CF population. One study demonstrated a significant response to **beta-agonists** at some point within a 12-month period in 95% of patients tested and showed an increased incidence of reactivity during acute exacerbations of the disease. At least some of the airway hyperreactivity is caused by secretions and edema in the airway wall rather than by smooth muscle hyperresponsiveness per se. The presence of airway hyperreactivity, as defined by a methacholine challenge test at a time of no clinical obstruction, correlates with a more rapid decline in pulmonary function. It is reasonable to advocate the use of beta-agonists in those patients with CF who wheeze clinically, demonstrate a significant bronchodilator response to beta-agonists, or have a positive methacholine challenge test, although routine methacholine challenge testing is not recommended.

Sputum in CF has increased viscosity because of increased glycoprotein sulfation and the presence of DNA released from dead leukocytes. With the exception of recombinant human deoxyribonuclease, mucolytic agents are not effective in CF. N-acetylcysteine administered by aerosol for inhalation may cause bronchospasm and is not recommended in these patients. Long-term beneficial effects of routine treatment with prednisone or nonsteroidal anti-inflammatory agents have not been demonstrated convincingly.

The present patient was treated at home using oxygen, aerosolized albuterol, prednisolone, parenteral nutrition, intravenous antibiotics, chest physical therapy, and pulmonary toilet. He improved and resumed normal activities.

Clinical Pearls

1. Airway hyperreactivity is present in 50–60% of patients with cystic fibrosis.
2. The use of beta adrenergic agonists is advocated in patients with cystic fibrosis who demonstrate clinical symptoms suggestive of bronchoconstriction.
3. The primary goal in the care of the pediatric patient with cystic fibrosis is to prevent infection and support nutrition.

REFERENCES

1. Konig P, Gayer D, Barbero GJ, Shaffer J. Short-term and long-term effects of albuterol aerosol therapy in cystic fibrosis: A preliminary report. Pediatr Pulmonol 1995;20:205–214.
2. de Jong W, Grevink RG, Roorda RJ. Effect of a home exercise training program in patients with cystic fibrosis. Chest 1994;105:463–468.
3. Konstan M, Stern R, Doershuk C. Efficacy of the flutter device for airway mucus clearance in patients with cystic fibrosis. J Pediatr 1994;124:689–693.
4. Marshall SG, Ramsey BW. Aerosol therapy in cystic fibrosis: DNase, tobramycin. Semin Respir Crit Care Med 1994;15:434–438.
5. Eggleston P, Rosenstein B, Stackhouse C. Airway hyperreactivity in cystic fibrosis: Clinical correlates and possible effects on the course of the disease. Chest 1988;94:360–365.

PATIENT 66

A 7-year-old boy with increasing weakness, a fading voice, and dysphagia

A 67-year-old boy was evaluated at his physician's office for increasing weakness, a fading voice, and dysphagia of 2-week duration. He had several recent, unexplained falls and difficulty swallowing.

Physical Examination: Temperature 98.6°; pulse 130; respirations 40; blood pressure 116/72. Chest: diminished breath sounds bilaterally. Cardiac: normal. Abdomen: normal. Extremities: without clubbing or edema. Neurologic: alert and oriented; cranial nerves—diminished gag, bilateral ptosis; motor—3–4/5 strength in proximal muscle groups; sensory intact; deep tendon reflexes absent.

Laboratory Findings: ABG (room air): pH 7.35, pCO_2 43 mmHg, pO_2 82 mmHg, HCO_3^- 22 mEq/L, SaO_2 96%. PFT: FVC 300 ml, NIF –18 cm H_2O, Vt_{spont} 55–80 ml. Chest radiograph (see below): no acute infiltrates.

Questions: What likely explains the boy's weakness? What are the implications of his illness on respiratory function?

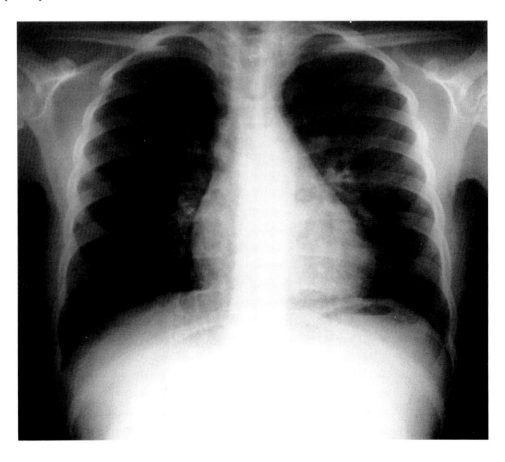

Diagnosis: Duchenne's muscular dystrophy.

Discussion: Duchenne's muscular dystrophy (DMD) is an X-linked recessive trait that affects approximately 1 in 3,500 male births. The abnormal gene causes the absence or malfunction of the **protein dystrophin** in skeletal muscle. Though histopathologic evidence of myopathy in patients with DMD is present soon after birth, the onset of clinically apparent muscle weakness, manifest by toe-walking and frequent falling episodes, usually is between the ages of 2 and 3. Children may not receive medical evaluation until proximal muscle weakness is sufficiently severe to cause difficulty ambulating. In the usual pattern of disease, proximal muscle weakness occurs first, but eventually all skeletal muscle groups will be involved. Deep tendon reflexes are diminished or absent.

The decline in muscular strength is linear throughout childhood; however, the severity of weakness may vary widely in children of similar ages. At 3–8 years, the child displays progressive contracture of the Achilles tendon, a more pronounced unsteady gait, and increased toe-walking. As the gait becomes more precarious, the child falls more often. Functional activity declines rapidly after 8 years of age due to increasing muscle weakness and contracture. The child usually is wheelchair-bound by the age of 12; some children remain ambulatory for a bit longer. The manifestation of respiratory symptoms is of particular concern. Deterioration of vital capacity to < 20% of normal leads to symptoms of nocturnal hypoventilation.

Although DMD is not curable, there is evidence that treatment with **corticosteroids** may have a beneficial effect on the natural history of the disease. Also, **physical therapy** can serve to maintain function, prevent contractures, and provide psychological support for the child and family. Efforts should be made to keep the patient ambulatory as long as possible, as quality of life is preserved with self-initiated ambulation.

The major morbidity and mortality in this disease is related to **respiratory failure**. Because of the skeletal muscle weakness, maximal inspiratory pressures are decreased at all lung volumes, and forced vital capacity begins to decline severely by the time patients are wheelchair-bound. Respiratory drive seems intact; however, hypercapnia generally is countered by increasing respiratory rate, rather than by tidal volume, as in normal subjects. **Scoliosis**, which often develops as a result of weakness of the paraspinal musculature, contributes to the respiratory muscle dysfunction. The scoliosis may add to the restrictive impairment and lead to inefficient use of respiratory muscles, thereby aggravating the effect of the dystrophy.

With the invariable decline in respiratory muscle strength, otherwise innocuous intercurrent illnesses such as the development of lobar pneumonia, atelectasis, or even abdominal distension associated with an ileus may lead to acute respiratory failure from which recovery may be poor. When respiratory failure has become permanent, options for ventilation include negative-pressure ventilation with a cuirass or other approach, or intermittent positive-pressure breathing with a noninvasive method such as a nasal mask. The decision to perform a tracheostomy to allow permanent positive-pressure breathing is a difficult one that should be made only after long and frank discussions with the patient and family.

The present patient was treated with an empiric course of prednisolone, and his respiratory mechanics were monitored at home. Hospitalization was not required.

Clinical Pearls

1. The incidence of Duchenne's muscular dystrophy is 1 in 3,500 male births.
2. CO_2 retention progresses in proportion to the severity of respiratory muscle weakness.
3. The immediate cause of death in Duchenne's muscular dystrophy is not always clear; however, respiratory insufficiency is a contributing factor in almost every patient.

REFERENCES

1. Rideau Y, Delaubier A, Guillou C, Renardel-Irani A. Treatment of respiratory insufficiency in Duchenne's muscular dystrophy: Nasal ventilation in the initial stages. Monaldi Arch Chest Dis 1995;50:235–238.
2. Lyager S, Steffensen B, Juhl B. Indicators of need for mechanical ventilation in Duchenne muscular dystrophy and spinal muscular atrophy. Chest 1995;108:779–785.
3. Backman E, Henriksson KG. Low-dose prednisolone treatment in Duchenne and Becker muscular dystrophy. Neuromuscul Disord 1995;5:233–241.
4. Chalmers RM, Howard RS, Wiles CM, Spencer GT. Use of the rocking bed in the treatment of neurogenic respiratory insufficiency. Q J M 1994;87:423–429.

PATIENT 67

A 34-year-old woman with fever, chills, and increased sputum production

A 34-year-old woman was seen in the emergency department for fever, chills, and increased sputum production of 2-day duration. Medical history included asthma and bronchitis. She had a 36-pack-year smoking history. Medications included albuterol, salmeterol, and oral contraceptives.

Physical Examination: Temperature 100.4°; pulse 76; respirations 32; blood pressure 150/88. Chest: bilateral rhonchi and wheezes with poor air entry. Cardiac: regular rhythm without murmurs. Abdomen: without organomegaly. Extremities: no cyanosis, clubbing, or edema. Neurologic: alert and oriented, nonfocal.

Laboratory Findings: WBC 12,990/μl, Hct 34.7%. ABG (non-rebreathing mask): pH 7.34, pCO_2 52 mmHg, pO_2 119 mmHg, HCO_3^- 21 mEq/L, SaO_2 97%. Chest radiograph (see below): revealed right middle and right lower lobe infiltrates.

Hospital Course: The patient was intubated to control and protect the airway and placed on mechanical ventilatory support. Upon intubation, the patient was noted to have peak airway pressures in excess of 50 cm H_2O, and copious secretions were suctioned from the endotracheal tube.

Question: What is the best approach to secretion control in this patient?

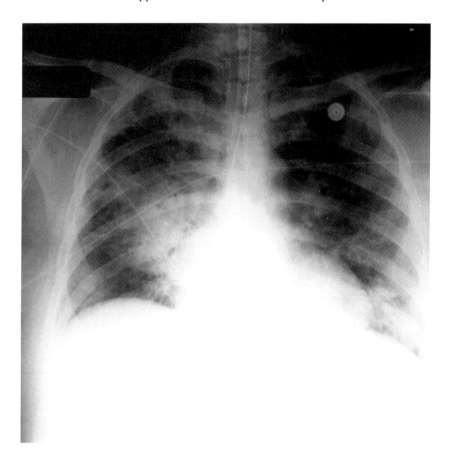

Diagnosis: Bacterial pneumonia.

Discussion: Control of airway secretions is a major respiratory care concern in patients receiving mechanical ventilation. Secretions may obstruct the patient's bronchi, causing atelectasis and worsening ventilation/perfusion (V/Q) mismatch, and may block the endotracheal tube itself, causing high airway pressures. Because of their inability to effectively mobilize secretions, all patients with artificial airways require **airway suctioning**. Additionally, the mouth and oral pharynx must be periodically suctioned because they can become reservoirs for microorganisms as a result of swallowing difficulties, especially when endotracheal tubes are in place. Suctioning should not be performed on a scheduled basis, as the procedure has potentially serious side effects, but rather should be prompted by the presence of secretions in the airway upon physical examination.

Hypoxemia has long been recognized as a potential hazard of airway suctioning. Factors which predispose the patient to hypoxemia during the suctioning procedure include interruption of oxygenation, breaking positive end-expiratory pressure (PEEP), and interrupting mechanical ventilation; aspiration of gas from the respiratory tract; entrainment of room air into the lungs; and prolonged duration of the procedure with the development of atelectasis. The best method of preventing the hypoxemia associated with suctioning is to hyperoxygenate the patient before and after the procedure. This is accomplished with either a hand-held resuscitator with PEEP as necessary, or by using the mechanical ventilator and making suitable adjustments for FiO_2 and flow rate. **Bradyarrhythmias**, the most common arrhythmias seen during the suctioning procedure, usually result from hypoxemia or vagal stimulation. However, more serious arrhythmias have been observed, including ventricular fibrillation and ventricular tachycardia with cardiac arrest.

Problems with tissue trauma and atelectasis can be avoided by using an appropriately sized and designed suction catheter, properly setting vacuum pressure, and applying expert technique. The suction catheter should be no larger than one-half the internal diameter of the artificial airway. The catheter should be long enough to enter the mainstem bronchi (22 inches long), have a means to interrupt vacuum (usually a thumb port), be flexible enough to prevent damage to the delicate mucosa but rigid enough to allow passage through the artificial airway, have smooth molded ends to prevent airway mucosal damage, and be capable of effectively removing mucus at a pressure that does not damage the tracheal or oropharyngeal mucosa. Suction pressure should be regulated to minimize the risk of atelectasis and still be effective. Proper technique includes a gentle but quick insertion and advancement of the catheter to its maximum length without suction being applied. Then while the catheter is removed slowly using a rotating motion, suction is applied intermittently.

Suctioning of patients receiving mechanical ventilatory support can be accomplished while the patient is connected to the mechanical ventilator or while disconnected briefly. Patients generally tolerate the off-ventilator technique well, whether the reoxygenation between passes of the catheter is provided by a manual resuscitator or by the ventilator itself. For patients who remain connected to the ventilator and are treated by a method of closed-system suction, heightened clinician awareness is essential. A suction catheter inserted into a closed-system circuit acts as an obstruction to ventilation and may exacerbate the complications of the suctioning procedure itself.

An effective, comprehensive program for preventing infection and controlling the potential risks associated with suctioning procedures entails universal precautions. Aseptic technique involving sterile gloves and suction catheters and rinsing solutions is recommended for any airway-related suction procedure.

Approaches not likely to benefit patients with secretions include the routine administration of mucolytic agents such as n-acetylcysteine and routine fiberoptic bronchoscopy with suctioning. Neither of these approaches provides benefits in addition to those achieved with the procedures described above.

The present patient was treated with combination antibiotic therapy for pneumonia. Bronchopulmonary hygiene was continued. Asthma symptoms were controlled and she was extubated on day 4.

Clinical Pearls

1. Because complications associated with suctioning are common (though often unrecognized), the procedure should be performed only as needed, not according to a preset schedule.

2. Suction should *never* be applied to the airway while the catheter is being inserted. This predisposes the patient to hypoxemia, atelectasis, and tissue trauma.

3. When suctioning patients, vacuum regulator settings of 120–150 mmHg are suitable for adults, 100–120 mmHg are suitable for children, and 80–100 mmHg are suitable for infants.

REFERENCES

1. Lebowitz LC, Mazzagatti FA. Comments on closed-system suction catheters. Respir Care 1995;40:1076–1077.
2. Copnell B, Fergusson D. Endotracheal suctioning: Time-worn ritual or timely intervention? Am J Crit Care 1995;4:100–105.
3. American Association for Respiratory Care. Clinical practice guideline: Endotracheal suctioning of mechanically ventilated adults and children with artificial airways. Respir Care 1993;38:500–504.
4. Mancinelli-Van Atta J, Beck SL. Preventing hypoxemia and hemodynamic compromise related to endotracheal suctioning. Am J Crit Care 1992;1:62–79.
5. Walsh JM, Vanderwarf C, Hoscheit D, et al. Unsuspected hemodynamic alterations during endotracheal suctioning. Chest 1989;95:162–165.

PATIENT 68

A 29-year-old woman with progressive productive cough, anorexia, and fever

A 29-year-old woman, a recent immigrant from Mexico now living in New York City and 27 weeks pregnant, came to the emergency department because of progressive productive cough of several weeks' duration, malaise, and fever. She reported that her sputum had been scanty and whitish yellow and that for 3 days it contained flecks of blood.

Physical Examination: Temperature 100.3°; pulse 85; respirations 18; blood pressure 142/88. Chest: dullness to percussion with rhonchi and bronchial breath sounds over the left middle and upper lung fields. Cardiac: regular rate and rhythm. Abdomen: normal for 26–28 weeks' gestation. Extremities: without cyanosis or clubbing. Neurologic: normal.

Laboratory Findings: CBC and electrolytes were within normal limits. SpO_2 (room air): 94%. Chest radiograph (see below): consolidation to the right middle and upper lobes.

Question: What is the most likely diagnosis in this patient?

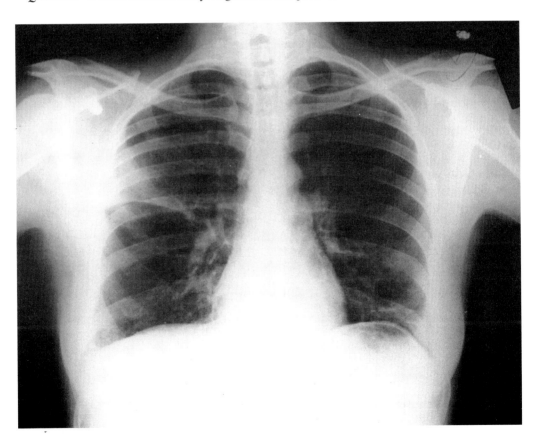

Diagnosis: Pulmonary tuberculosis in a pregnant patient.

Discussion: Though the incidence of tuberculosis in the United States as a whole is less than 9 per 100,000 cases, in inner cities and other urban areas it may be five to six times higher. Persons at greatest risk for tuberculosis in the United States include those with human immunodeficiency virus (HIV) infection, intravenous drug users, those of lower socioeconomic status, and recent immigrants from countries with a high prevalence of tuberculosis, such as Africa, Asia, and parts of Central and South America. The complaints of fever and chronic cough in any person with these characteristics should prompt a diagnostic evaluation for tuberculosis. In addition, patients with advanced malignancy, end stage renal disease, diabetes mellitus, silicosis, malnutrition, or who are taking immunosuppressive drugs such as azathioprine or high doses of corticosteroids also are at risk for tuberculosis. HIV testing should be strongly encouraged in most newly diagnosed patients with tuberculosis in the United States.

Chest radiographic findings typical of tuberculosis are **upper lobe infiltrates**, which may cavitate. Other radiographic presentations, such as pleural effusion or lower lobe disease (the latter particularly in patients with diabetes), also may be seen. In persons with severe immunodeficiency (such as advanced HIV infection), mediastinal lymphadenopathy may be the sole radiographic finding. When the diagnosis is suspected, sputum examination for acid-fast bacillus (AFB) is the next diagnostic step. If the AFB smear is positive, therapy should be started immediately. However, smears will be positive only in 50–75% of tuberculosis cases, so a negative smear does not exclude the diagnosis if the clinical suspicion is high. Presumptive therapy should be given until culture results and clinical response to treatment can be evaluated.

Tuberculosis in a pregnant woman raises several important considerations. Most recent evidence suggests that pregnant women with latent tuberculosis are no more likely to develop active tuberculosis after becoming pregnant than they were before. In addition, the outcome of a pregnancy in a woman with properly treated tuberculosis should be no different than in a pregnancy not complicated by tuberculosis. However, **newborn infants are extremely susceptible** to tuberculosis infection, and it is clear that the benefits of treating a pregnant woman (both for her and for her baby) far outweigh the risks to the developing fetus. Isoniazid, rifampin, and ethambutol are all safe in pregnancy and should be started in any pregnant woman with tuberculosis. Less information is available on pyrazinamide, and its routine use is not recommended in the U.S. during pregnancy. The medications can be adjusted when drug susceptibility results are available.

The primary goal in treating the pregnant woman with tuberculosis is to render the AFB smear negative at the time of delivery. If the patient is still infectious at the time of delivery, the newborn may have to be separated from the mother until she is no longer infectious. If separation is impossible, vaccination with bacille Calmette-Guérin may be indicated—but should be undertaken only in consultation with the local health department.

There is some evidence that women in the peripartum stage are more likely to develop isoniazid-related hepatitis than non-pregnant women, so tuberculosis therapy given during and just after pregnancy should be monitored with monthly liver function tests.

The present patient had positive sputum smear for AFB and was started on anti-tuberculous chemotherapy. Her symptoms improved within 2 weeks and, taking medication throughout her pregnancy, she had an uncomplicated course with delivery of a healthy infant. She completed her tuberculosis therapy after delivery.

Clinical Pearls

1. Isoniazid, rifampin, and ethambutol remain the cornerstones of therapy for pregnant patients with active tuberculosis.

2. The benefits of treating active tuberculosis in a pregnant woman far outweigh the risks to the woman or developing fetus.

3. The risk of isoniazid-related hepatitis may be high in the peripartum period, and patients receiving medication during this time should be monitored with monthly liver function tests.

REFERENCES

1. Margono F, Mroueh J, Garely A. Resurgence of active tuberculosis among pregnant women. Obstet Gynecol 1994;83:911–914.
2. Carter EJ, Mates S. Tuberculosis during pregnancy: The Rhode Island experience 1987–1991. Chest 1994;106:1466–1470.
3. Margono F, Garely A, Mroueh J. Tuberculosis among pregnant women, New York City 1985–1992. MMWR 1993;42:605–612.

PATIENT 69

A 77-year-old woman with acute respiratory distress while on mechanical ventilation

A 77-year-old woman being ventilated for acute pulmonary edema was suddenly found to be tachypneic, coughing violently, and experiencing elevated peak airway pressures from the ventilator. Immediately prior to the patient's change in status, routine airway maintenance had been performed, including endotracheal suctioning and the changing of the tube tape.

Physical Examination: Temperature 98.9°; pulse 86; respirations 30; blood pressure 138/86. Chest: diminished breath sounds on the left. Cardiac: tachycardic. Abdomen: without organomegaly. Extremities: no cyanosis or edema. Neurologic: agitated, otherwise normal.

Laboratory Findings: WBC 8700/μl, Hct 50.8%. PT 10.9 sec, PTT 32 sec. PETCO$_2$ 26 mmHg, Paw 72 cmH$_2$O. ABG (FiO$_2$ .30): pH 7.59, pCO$_2$ 28 mmHg, pO$_2$ 71 mmHg, HCO$_3^-$ 32 mEq/L, SaO$_2$ 95%. Chest radiograph (see below): pulmonary vascular congestion.

Questions: What is the most likely cause of the change in the patient's clinical status? What is the significance of the end-tidal CO$_2$ reading?

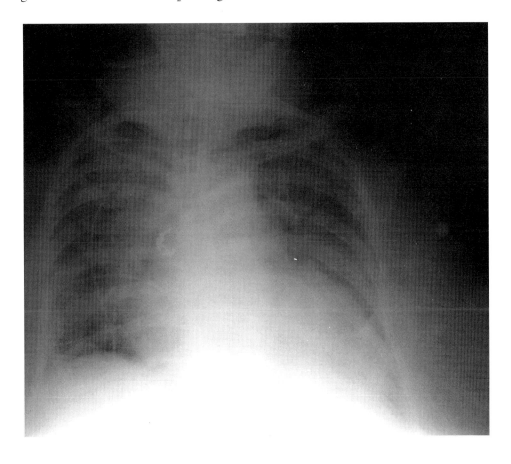

Diagnosis: Malposition of the endotracheal tube following airway care.

Discussion: Maintenance of artificial airways includes positioning, repositioning, and securing the tube; suctioning the airway; and monitoring tracheal cuff pressure with adjustments of intracuff volume and pressure. Almost any intervention in the patient with an artificial airway can have a deleterious effect on the integrity of that airway. Hazards include accidental extubation or decannulation, migration of the distal end of the tube into a main stem bronchus (most often the right), over- or underinflation of the cuff, and creation of subglottic edema. *Extreme caution* must be exercised for every procedure performed on a patient with an artificial airway that may involve breaching the integrity of the tube and ventilator circuit.

During mechanical ventilatory support, confirmation of oxygenation and ventilation remains an important component of total patient monitoring. While arterial blood gases have been the traditional gold standard for the detection of hypoxemia and hypercapnia, noninvasive means of monitoring respiratory data are becoming more widely used and accepted. **Capnography**, which displays CO_2 concentration changes during the respiratory cycle, allows noninvasive, rapid identification of problems such as esophageal intubation, inadvertent bronchial intubation, and apnea.

Two techniques may be used for capnography: mass spectroscopy and infrared absorption. Variables such as response time, number of patients to be analyzed, and equipment availability suggest which technique is appropriate. As a practical matter, it is important to remember that the circuitry used to measure end-tidal CO_2 may add significantly to the dead space of the ventilator circuitry and have a negative impact on the patient in terms of overall ventilation.

In a normal lung, CO_2 rapidly diffuses across the alveolar-capillary membrane when ventilation and perfusion units are well matched. End-tidal CO_2 (PET_{CO_2}), defined as the partial pressure of CO_2 at the end of a tidal breath, closely approximates the arterial pCO_2 ($PaCO_2$) in normal lungs. In abnormal lungs, such as in underlying pulmonary disease, ventilation/perfusion ratios, total CO_2 production rates, and total alveolar ventilation may not be stable. As a rule the PET_{CO_2} tends to underestimate the $PaCO_2$, and for that reason the techniques may be insensitive to hypercapnia. Therefore, monitoring PET_{CO_2} alone may not be a reliable indicator during weaning or adjustments of mechanical ventilation, and, in general, capnography has limited utility in patients with cardiopulmonary disease, particularly in disease states characterized by ventilation/perfusion inequality.

Capnography may be used clinically in the following ways: to ensure the placement of an endotracheal tube, as an estimate of $PaCO_2$ in stable patients with normal systemic and pulmonary perfusion (such as patients undergoing elective surgery), as a reflection of a change in pulmonary blood flow or dead space ventilation, and to detect the addition of excess CO_2 to the systemic circulation. In terms of values, PET_{CO_2} is always less than or equal to $PaCO_2$ due to the exhaled gas contributed from ventilated but poorly perfused alveoli.

Physical examination in this patient suggested a right main bronchus intubation that occurred during manipulation of the endotracheal tube. Bronchial intubation was confirmed by chest radiograph. The tube was repositioned and the patient's respiratory status improved.

Clinical Pearls

1. Even routine airway care is associated with hazards for the patient, and the patient's respiratory status should be reassessed following every manipulation of the ventilator circuitry.

2. While capnography provides a means to evaluate the stability of ventilation, it usually underestimates the true $PaCO_2$ and also can underestimate the degree of hypercapnia.

3. Capnography is unreliable in patients with cardiopulmonary disease characterized by significant ventilation/perfusion imbalance.

REFERENCES

1. Palmon SC, Liu M, Moore LE, Kirsch JR. Capnography facilitates tight control of ventilation during transport. Crit Care Med 1996;24:608–611.
2. Stock MC. Capnography for adults. Crit Care Clin 1995;11:219–232.
3. Coaldrake LA. Capnography does not always indicate successful intubation. Anaesth Intensive Care 1995;23:616–617.
4. Spencer RF, Rathmell JP, Viscomi CM. A new method for difficult endotracheal intubation: The use of a jet stylet introducer and capnography. Anesth Analg 1995;81:1079–1083.
5. Sessler CN, Glass C, Grap MJ. Techniques for preventing and managing unplanned extubation. J Crit Illness 1994;9:609–619.
6. Truwit JD, Rochester DF. Monitoring the respiratory system of the mechanically ventilated patient. New Horiz 1994;2:94–106.

PATIENT 70

An 80-year-old woman with dyspnea, tachypnea, and chills

An 80-year-old woman was brought to the emergency department complaining of difficulty breathing, chills, and increased sputum production. Medical history included chronic obstructive pulmonary disease, hypertension, and coronary artery disease. She had a 63 pack-year cigarette smoking history. Medications included ranitidine, amlodipine, oxycodone/acetaminophen, theophylline, ipratropium, albuterol, and prednisolone.

Physical Examination: Temperature 99.3°; pulse 84; respirations 26; blood pressure 154/74. Chest: end-expiratory wheezing. Cardiac: regular rhythm. Abdomen: soft, without organomegaly. Extremities: no cyanosis or edema. Neurologic: alert and oriented, nonfocal.

Laboratory Findings: Glucose 138 mg/dl, theophylline 7.1 μg/ml. ABG (room air): pH 7.36, pCO_2 55 mmHg, pO_2 53 mmHg, HCO_3^- 31 mEq/L, SaO_2 89%. Chest radiograph (see below): revealed left lower lobe infiltrate.

Questions: How much, if any, supplemental oxygen should be administered to the patient? How should it be administered?

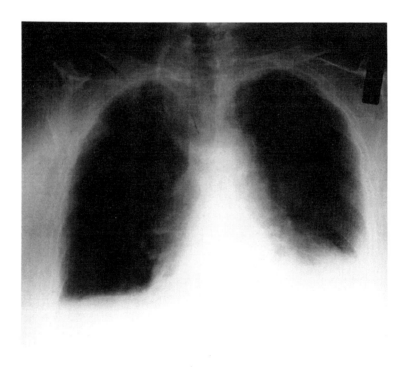

Diagnosis: Chronic obstructive pulmonary disease (COPD) exacerbation, with hypercapnic respiratory failure.

Discussion: Administration of oxygen to patients with COPD can be beneficial in the settings of both acute (as in this patient) and chronic respiratory failure. Indeed, **oxygen therapy** is the only therapeutic measure that has been demonstrated to prolong life in patients with COPD. Bronchodilator therapy, anti-inflammatory treatment, and antibiotics may all serve to improve symptoms, but they have no effect on the disease process itself. However, it has been convincingly demonstrated that in patients with COPD and chronically low pO_2 (below 55 mmHg), long-term oxygen therapy confers a survival benefit.

In the setting of an acute COPD exacerbation, supplemental oxygen therapy is aimed at boosting the pO_2 above 60 mmHg so that the patient can move to the flat portion of the oxyhemoglobin dissociation curve and be provided with a margin of safety. However, excessive oxygen administration in susceptible patients, primarily those with an acute worsening of chronic hypercapnia, can lead to acute-on-chronic hypercapnia and severe respiratory acidosis. Although the mechanism behind this **oxygen-induced hypercapnia** is not entirely clear, the importance of the observation is undeniable. Many a patient has been pushed into worse respiratory acidosis, often requiring intubation, by overzealous administration of oxygen.

Regarding the cause of oxygen-induced hypercapnia, for many years, it was thought that the hypoxic drive in patients with COPD played a prominent role in regulating minute ventilation, since chronic hypercapnia blunted the usual CO_2 stimulus to ventilation. It was further believed that supplemental oxygen suppressed the hypoxic drive and promoted hypercapnia in the setting of a reduced CO_2 response. More recent investigations have demonstrated that despite the occurrence of arterial hypercapnia, resting minute ventilation is maintained in hypercapnic COPD patients after the administration of supplemental oxygen. Therefore, if the $PaCO_2$ increases after the administration of supplemental oxygen without a change in minute ventilation, then a change in dead space ventilation/total ventilation (V_D/V_t) is present. This could be explained by a changing ventilation/perfusion (V/Q) relationship in response to oxygen administration without a significant extinguishing of the hypoxic drive to breathe. Currently, worsening V/Q imbalance is accepted as the major physiologic explanation behind oxygen-induced hypercapnia in patients with COPD.

Oxygen therapy is divided into two broad categories: high flow and low flow systems. **High flow systems** include any device capable of providing gas flow that either meets or exceeds the patient's peak inspiratory flow demand. These systems provide a precise and consistent FiO_2 independent of changes in the patient's depth, pattern, and rate of breathing. In essence, systems classified as high flow for adults (Venturi) must be capable of delivering at least 40 liters per minute of conditioned gas to the patient.

Low flow systems (nasal cannula, simple mask, partial rebreathing mask, and non-rebreathing mask) are devices in which the FiO_2 is dependent on the flow of oxygen into the device, the size of the reservoir, the capability of filling the reservoir between expiration and inspiration, and the ventilatory pattern of the patient. Because all of these factors determine FiO_2, it is virtually impossible to predict the precise FiO_2 that the patient is receiving with low flow systems.

When deciding which oxygen delivery system should be used in patients with acute exacerbation of COPD, the following questions are generally useful in guiding selection: What FiO_2 is needed? Are consistency and accuracy of FiO_2 required? Is tolerance and compliance a problem? Some clinicians prefer the use of Venturi masks in patients with COPD exacerbation. These masks provide precise delivery of oxygen at concentrations as low as 24 to 28%.

The present patient responded favorably to a high flow, low concentration 31% Venturi mask. Antibiotics were administered and her theophylline level was therapeutically regulated. She improved and was discharged.

Clinical Pearls

1. Supplemental oxygen given to patients with chronic obstructive pulmonary disease and acute hypercapnic respiratory failure can cause worsening hypercapnic and respiratory acidosis primarily by increasing ventilation/perfusion mismatching.

2. In a low flow oxygen system, the delivered FiO_2 is inversely proportional to the patient's minute ventilation.

3. A properly adjusted high flow system (such as a Venturi mask) ensures delivery of the selected FiO_2 by providing gas flow in excess of the patient's peak inspiratory flow demand.

REFERENCES

1. Hanson CW 3rd, Marshall BE, Frasch HF, Marshall C. Causes of hypercarbia with oxygen therapy in patients with chronic obstructive pulmonary disease. Crit Care Med 1996;24:23–82.
2. Tarpy SP, Celli BR. Long-term oxygen therapy. N Engl J Med 1995;333:710–714.
3. Costello RW, Liston R, McNicholas WT. Compliance at night with low flow oxygen therapy: A comparison of nasal cannulae and Venturi face masks. Thorax 1995;50:405–406.
4. American Association for Respiratory Care. Clinical practice guideline: Oxygen therapy in the acute care hospital. Respir Care 1991;36:1410–1413.

PATIENT 71

A 63-year-old man with chronic hypersensitivity pneumonitis and marked hypoxemia

A 63-year-old man was admitted to a medical floor with worsening shortness of breath of 5-day duration. He had a history of chronic hypersensitivity pneumonitis with extensive fibrosis, related to his occupation as a furrier. Medications included metaproterenol, salmeterol, and prednisolone.

Physical Examination: Temperature 100.2°; pulse 96; respirations 32; blood pressure 156/92. Chest: diminished breath sounds with expiratory wheezes. Cardiac: no murmurs. Abdomen: nontender, without masses or organomegaly. Extremities: peripheral cyanosis with clubbing. Neurologic: nonfocal.

Laboratory Findings: WBC 10,700/µl, Hct 49%. ABG (room air): pH 7.37, pCO_2 54 mmHg, pO_2 50 mmHg, HCO_3^- 30 mEq/L, SaO_2 77%. Chest radiograph (see below): interstitial fibrosis with narrow mediastinum.

Hospital Course: The patient was given supplemental oxygen which improved his oxygen saturation to 90%.

Question: What are the risks and benefits of long-term oxygen therapy?

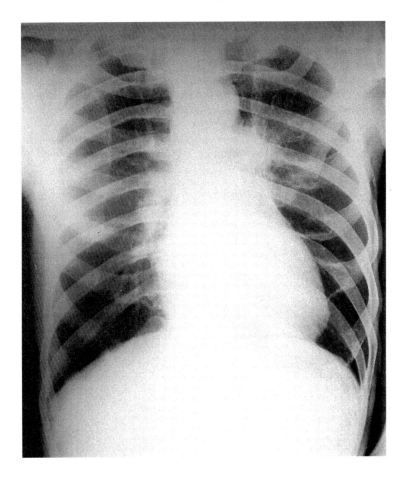

Diagnosis: End-stage lung disease due to chronic hypersensitivity pneumonitis, with hypoxic respiratory failure.

Discussion: The therapeutic value of supplemental oxygen breathing for clinical conditions characterized by hypoxemia is widely recognized. The use of oxygen is not without potential harm and the risks of high oxygen tensions should be appreciated.

The **adverse effects of oxygen therapy** can be categorized into alterations of normal physiology and direct cytotoxic effects. Supplemental oxygen can cause a variety of extrapulmonary toxicities. Retrolental fibroplasia may occur in neonates when they are exposed to hyperoxia. Seizures, paralysis, and myopia can occur during hyperbaric oxygen therapy. The hematopoietic system may be affected, possibly leading to depressed erythropoiesis. High oxygen tensions can cause decreased cardiac output and systemic vasoconstriction as well.

The **pulmonary** effects of hyperoxia include desiccation of the mucous membranes (if the gas is not adequately humidified), depression of ventilation, reversal of (compensatory) hypoxic pulmonary vasoconstriction, and absorption atelectasis. In patients with chronic obstructive lung disease (COPD), oxygen therapy can result in hypercapnia and precipitate respiratory failure. This phenomenon may in part be explained by an overreliance on hypoxic respiratory drive in the face of chronically elevated CO_2, which blunts the normal ventilatory response to CO_2. Oxygen therapy may also alter ventilation/perfusion (V/Q) ratios in patients with COPD, resulting in hypercapnia. Normally, the pulmonary vascular bed vasoconstricts in response to hypoxia to preserve V/Q matching.

Absorption atelectasis can occur when high oxygen tensions are instituted. Nitrogen is an inert gas that is normally located in the alveoli and acts as a physiologic stint. Alveolar nitrogen reserves may be washed out under conditions of high oxygen tensions. Subsequent absorption of alveolar oxygen in areas of the lung that are poorly ventilated results in absorption atelectasis. Consequently there is a decrease in vital capacity and an increase in pulmonary shunting, which may further decrease the arterial oxygen tension. Surfactant formation can also be impaired during hyperoxic exposure, further exacerbating this condition.

The **cytotoxic** effects of oxygen toxicity include tracheobronchitis, acute respiratory distress syndrome (ARDS), and bronchopulmonary dysplasia. Both tracheobronchitis and ARDS can result from breathing 100% oxygen (and in experimental models, oxygen toxicity can occur with FiO_2 as low as .5, if given for a prolonged period) with tracheobronchitis beginning as early as 12–24 hours after exposure. Dry cough and substernal chest pain, often with a pleuritic component, signal the onset of tracheobronchitis. Symptoms at 24–36 hours include paresthesias, nausea, vomiting, and headache. Protein synthesis may become impaired in endothelial cells, leading to faulty cell function. Lung compliance and diffusion capacity are reduced while the (A-a)DO_2 gradient increases. At 48–60 hours, surfactant production is inactivated and alveolar edema occurs. Finally, at 60 hours, histologic changes of the pulmonary parenchyma become overtly evident as ARDS progresses. Respiratory failure and death may ensue if 100% oxygen breathing continues.

The primary mechanism by which oxygen exerts its toxic effects is through the generation of oxygen free radicals. The free-radical theory of oxygen toxicity states that during exposure to increased partial pressures of oxygen, an increased rate of generation of partially reduced oxygen products results in cell damage. The oxygen molecule itself is relatively nonreactive and does not lead to direct tissue injury. However, normal metabolic processes generate small amounts of superoxide anion (O_2^-) and hydrogen peroxide (H_2O_2), the one- and two-electron reduction products of molecular oxygen. These primary products can lead to the formation of the per-hydroxy and hydroxyl radicals, which are the most reactive and damaging O_2-derived products.

The cytotoxic effect of superoxide anion and other oxygen-derived radicals originate from their interaction with key cellular components. Normally, cellular antioxidants maintain the cellular concentration of oxy radicals at low levels. Additionally, tissue reparative mechanisms restore oxidized cell components to their reduced state to prevent overt manifestations of cellular toxicity. With exposure to hyperoxia, the increased rate of radical generation overwhelms antioxidant defenses.

The present patient succumbed to refractory hypoxemia shortly after discharge.

Clinical Pearls

1. Pulmonary oxygen toxicity can be seen while breathing concentrations of oxygen greater than .5, although this is usually in the context of gas delivered via mechanical ventilation.

2. Although nitrogen in air theoretically acts as a physiologic stent, there is no evidence that oxygen/nitrogen mixtures prevent absorption atelectasis.

3. Tracheobronchitis can begin as early as 12–24 hours after the initiation of 100% oxygen.

REFERENCES

1. Kazzaz JA, Xu J, Palaia TA, et al. Cellular oxygen toxicity: Oxidant injury without apoptosis. J Biol Chem 1996;271: 15182–15186.
2. Jenkinson SG. Oxygen toxicity [Review]. New Horiz 1993;1:504–511.
3. Stogner SW, Payne DK. Oxygen toxicity. Ann Pharmacother 1992;26:1554–1562.
4. Griffith DE, Garcia JG, James HL, et al. Hyperoxic exposure in humans: Effects of 50% oxygen on alveolar macrophage leukotriene B4 synthesis. Chest 1992;101:392–397.

PATIENT 72

A 47-year-old man with renal failure, cyanosis, and sudden unresponsiveness

A 47-year-old obese man developed severe respiratory distress and cyanosis while undergoing hemodialysis. Medical history included hypertension, renal failure, and non–insulin-dependent diabetes mellitus. Medications included furosemide, glyburide, and lisinopril.

Physical Examination: Temperature 99.6°; pulse 128; respirations 28; blood pressure 160/110. Chest: clear, air entry poor. Cardiac: tachycardic. Abdomen: obese, nontender. Extremities: cyanotic. Neurologic: unresponsive.

Laboratory Findings: Na^+ 137 mEq/L, Cl^- 104 mEq/L, K^+ 5.8 mEq/L. HCO_3^- 11 mEq/L, TCO_2 14 mEq/L. Glucose 115 mg/dl, BUN 130 mg/dl, Cr 10 mg/dl. ABG (non-rebreathing mask): pH 7.27, pCO_2 25 mmHg, pO_2 62 mmHg, SaO_2 91%. Chest radiograph (see below): revealed left pleural effusion.

Hospital Course: Because of severe respiratory distress, intubation was attempted but not immediately achieved.

Question: How can a difficult airway be managed in an acute emergency?

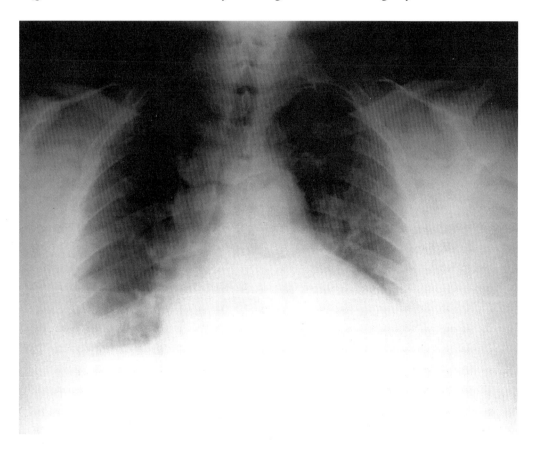

Answer/Discussion: Difficult intubation can occur unexpectedly in clinical practice. However, some cases may be foreseen. A **rapid assessment of the airway** should be performed when management decisions involve the maintenance of airway patency and gas exchange. A difficult airway is one in which there are problems with bag-and-mask ventilation or with laryngoscopy and tracheal intubation, or with both. The consequences of failed intubation can be devastating. Clinicians responsible for providing this aspect of care should know and follow a logical process intended to address this problem.

The problem of a difficult airway in a patient with respiratory failure may be more serious than in a patient presenting for elective surgery. First, the elective surgery patient can be awakened and the surgery postponed or cancelled while further evaluation is performed. Second, the elective surgery patient is less likely to have significant underlying pathology, whereas the patient with respiratory failure may have severe pulmonary pathology, hypercapnia, and desaturation. Third, higher airway resistance and lower pulmonary compliance are often present with respiratory failure, making bag-and-mask ventilation difficult to use as a temporary measure.

A rapid assessment is required before intubation attempts to determine the likelihood of a difficult intubation. The assessment begins with an examination of facial anatomy from frontal and lateral views. This examination serves to identify any gross deviations from normal (prognathia, retrognathia, overbite, or facial swelling).

In addition, if the patient can open his or her mouth and protrude the tongue, then the **Mallampati classification** system may be applied. It defines four classes of airway according to what structures are visible following protusion of the tongue. Class I allows visualization of the soft palate, fauces uvula, and anterior and posterior tonsillar pillars. Patients in this class typically have atraumatic, uneventful intubations. Class II allows visualization of the soft palate, fauces, and uvula. Class III allows visualization of the soft palate and the base of the uvula. Class IV disallows visualization of any respiratory structure with the exception of parts of the soft palate. Patients in this class are at risk for traumatic intubation due to nonvisualization of the vocal cords during laryngoscopy.

If initial intubation attempts fail but mask ventilation is *adequate*, options include further attempts at intubation using alternate laryngoscope blades, intubation with a bronchoscope, or other specialized procedure. If initial intubation attempts fail and mask ventilation is *inadequate*, the clinician should immediately call for help. In emergency intubation, the clinician must be familiar with alternatives for a patient with a difficult airway. Alternatives include but are not limited to nasotracheal intubation, fiberoptic intubation, use of a lighted stylet, retrograde intubation, and cricothyroidotomy. (In retrograde intubation, a flexible guide is inserted through a cricothyroid membrane and threaded caudad until it can be secured at the nose or mouth. An endotracheal tube then can be placed over the guide and positioned.) Needless to say, these techniques should be attempted only by trained personnel.

Muscle relaxants or rapid sequence intubation may assist in the establishment of an airway in this population of patients. An important caveat to remember in the use of paralyzing agents is that depolarizing agents such as succinylcholine can cause life-threatening hyperkalemia in patients with preexisting renal failure or neuromuscular disease. Also, the intubation operator must be highly skilled in intubation and face mask ventilation so as to support a paralyzed, apneic patient.

The present patient's airway was established using retrograde intubation, and mechanical ventilatory support was provided.

Clinical Pearls

1. Physicians who perform translaryngeal intubation should be knowledgeable in the techniques to evaluate and manage the difficult airway.

2. Succinylcholine should be avoided in patients with renal failure and neuromuscular disease because of the risks of inducing hyperkalemia.

3. A rapid facial and oral examination is the first step in intubation in order to assess the likelihood of a difficult intubation.

REFERENCES

1. Jacobsen J, Jensen E, Waldau T, Poulsen TD. Preoperative evaluation of intubation conditions in patients scheduled for elective surgery. Acta Anaesthesiol Scand 1996;40:421–424.
2. West MR, Jonas MM, Adams AP, Carli F. A new tracheal tube for difficult intubation. Brit J Anaesth 1996;76:673–679.
3. Benumof JL. Laryngeal mask airway and the ASA difficult airway algorithm. Anesthesiology 1996;84:686–699.
4. Schwartz DE, Matthay MA, Cohen NH. Death and other complications of emergency airway management in critically ill adults: A prospective investigation of 297 tracheal intubations. Anesthesiology 1995;82:367–376.
5. Deem S, Bishop MJ. Evaluation and management of the difficult airway. Crit Care Clin 1995;11:1–27.
6. Mazzagatti FA. Rapid sequence intubation. J Emerg Med Serv 1995;20:17–18.
7. American Society of Anesthesiologists Task Force. Practice guidelines for management of the difficult airway. Anesthesiology 1993;78:597–602.

PATIENT 73

**A 55-year-old man with dyspnea, fever, and dense consolidation
of the right lower lobe**

A 55-year-old man was brought to the emergency department with shaking chills, right-sided pleuritic chest pain, and a cough productive of thick bloody sputum. Medical history included binge drinking of alcohol. He denied taking any medications.

Physical Examination: Temperature 104.2°; pulse 104; respirations 29; blood pressure 120/55. HEENT: poor dentition. Chest: pleural friction rub to the right posterior thorax. Cardiac: no murmurs or gallops. Abdomen: nontender, without organomegaly. Extremities: no cyanosis or clubbing. Neurologic: alert.

Laboratory Findings: WBC 4,000/μl, Hct 36%, platelets 97,000/μl. Glucose 115 mg/dl. ABG (room air): pH 7.47, pCO_2 33 mmHg, pO_2 67 mmHg, HCO_3^- 27 mEq/L, SaO_2 93%. Gram stain (sputum): many polymorphonuclear neutrophils and plump gram-negative rods. Chest radiograph (see below): right lobar consolidation with volume loss.

Question: What is the most likely diagnosis in this patient?

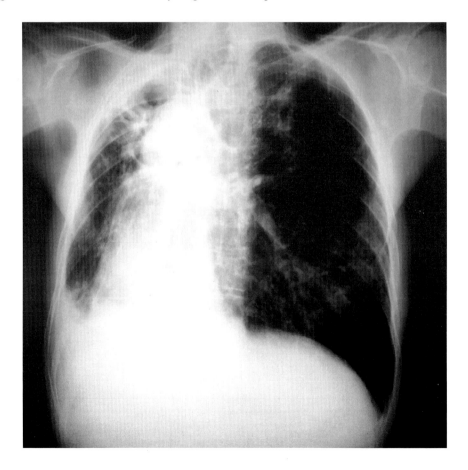

Diagnosis: *Klebsiella pneumoniae* pneumonia in an alcoholic.

Discussion: The diagnosis and treatment of community-acquired pneumonia remains one of the most common clinical problems in pulmonary medicine. In recent years, emphasis has shifted away from expensive and comprehensive diagnostic testing due to recognition that, despite intensive investigation, a specific etiologic agent is not identifiable for the majority of cases of community-acquired pneumonia. Furthermore, it is not clear that outcome is affected by the identification of a specific etiologic pathogen. Therapy should be guided by the presence of clinical and demographic factors associated with specific pathogens. Thus, for example, persons in the southwestern United States are at risk for coccidioidomycosis, while those in the Ohio River Valley are susceptible to histoplasmosis. Persons with poor dentition are prone to the development of anaerobic pneumonia. **Alcoholics**, in particular, while being susceptible to the usual pathogens such as *S. pneumoniae* and *H. influenzae*, also are prone to two other syndromes: lung abscess due to aspiration and acute pneumonia caused by *Klebsiella pneumoniae*.

Klebsiella pneumoniae is an encapsulated, nonmotile bacillus with an affinity for causing pneumonia in the right upper lobe. It produces an extensive, hemorrhagic, necrotizing consolidation of the lung that can be fatal. It most often affects middle-aged men, alcoholics, diabetics, the malnourished, and those with chronic obstructive pulmonary disease. The sputum can be thick, blood-stained, and tenacious and is sometimes described as "red currant jelly" in appearance.

Klebsiella pneumoniae accounts for less than one percent of all bacterial pneumonias, but remains the most common cause of community-acquired gram-negative pneumonias. Traditionally the clinical manifestations have been thought to present as two different syndromes: typical and atypical. The **typical pneumonia syndrome** is characterized by sudden onset of fever, productive cough, pleuritic chest pain, tactile fremitus, dullness to percussion, and egophony. The **atypical pneumonia syndrome** is characterized by a more gradual onset, dry cough, extrapulmonary symptoms (e.g., headache, myalgias, fatigue), and abnormalities on chest radiograph. Lobar consolidation is the rule and there may be evidence of volume loss due to mucous plugging from tenacious secretions. The classic chest radiograph, which shows lobar consolidation with a bulging fissure, occurs only occasionally.

Most strains of *Klebsiella pneumoniae* are sensitive to third generation cephalosporins and aminoglycosides and are naturally resistant to ampicillin and carbenicillin.

The present patient was treated with cefuroxime and amikacin and was discharged on the 10th day following admission.

Clinical Pearls

1. The diagnosis of *Klebsiella pneumoniae* pneumonia should be considered in patients presenting with respiratory symptoms who also have significant underlying disease such as diabetes, alcoholism, or chronic obstructive pulmonary disease.

2. Sputum associated with *Klebsiella pneumoniae* occasionally has a red currant jelly–like appearance, and the classical chest radiograph may reveal a bulging fissure.

3. Empiric antibiotic therapy in patients presenting with community-acquired pneumonia should be chosen to cover pathogens suggested by the patient's clinical characteristics and epidemiologic setting.

REFERENCES
1. Jong GM, Hsiue TR, Chen CR, et al. Rapidly fatal outcome of bacteremic *Klebsiella pneumoniae* pneumonia in alcoholics. Chest 1995;107:214–217.
2. Bartlett JG, Mundy LM: Community-acquired pneumonia. New Engl J Med 1995;333:1618–1624.
3. Niederman MS, Bass JB Jr, Campbell GD, et al: Guidelines for the initial management of adults with community-acquired pneumonia: Diagnosis, assessment of severity, and initial antimicrobial therapy. Am Rev Respir Dis 1993;148:1418–1426.

PATIENT 74

**A 29-year-old woman with paroxysmal nocturnal dyspnea
and orthopnea**

A 29-year-old woman presented to her physician complaining of nighttime coughing and dyspnea. Medical history included gastroesophageal reflux and childhood asthma. She had experienced no exacerbations of her asthma over the previous 15 years. Medications included aluminum/magnesium hydroxide with simethicone.

Physical Examination: Temperature 98.8; pulse 96; respirations 20; blood pressure 126/84. Chest: clear to auscultation. Cardiac: regular rhythm, without murmurs or gallops. Abdomen: nontender, without organomegaly. Neurologic: alert, oriented.

Laboratory Findings: ABG (room air): pH 7.53, pCO_2 32 mmHg, pO_2 87 mmHg, HCO_3^- 22 mEq/L, SaO_2 96%. Chest radiograph: see below.

Question: What are the likely causes of this patient's cough?

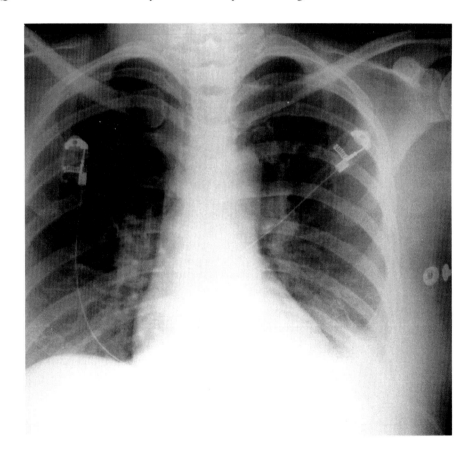

Diagnosis: Nocturnal asthma.

Discussion: Chronic cough, particularly a cough that occurs at night, usually is due to one of four problems: asthma (so-called cough-variant asthma), gastroesophageal reflux (GERD), post-nasal drip, and chronic sinusitis. The evaluation of chronic cough should always include **pulmonary function testing** (PFT), which demonstrates airflow obstruction in asthmatics. If PFT is normal (including a normal bronchoprovocation study), GERD and sinus disease should be investigated with a barium swallow (or perhaps a Bernstein test for acid reflux) and sinus films.

Nocturnal asthma, also referred to as sleep-related asthma, can be difficult to diagnose and treat. Patients complaining of asthma-related symptoms do not always identify the times at which their symptoms are more severe. Development of symptoms or decrements in airway function frequently occur in the asthmatic during sleep. Even in the normal patient, airway dynamics fluctuate between day and night. The best lung function typically occurs at 4 PM and the worst at 4 AM. The peak-to-trough difference can be as high as 50%.

Although the cause of nocturnal exacerbation of asthma is not thoroughly understood, a combination of multiple effects controls the airway of the susceptible patient. These processes include the net effect that catecholamines, beta-adrenergic receptor responsiveness, mucociliary clearance, reflux mechanisms, vagal tone, inflammatory cells/mediators, corticosteroids, immunologic integrity, and arousal patterns have on airway dynamics. The circadian rhythms of all these variables appear to be arranged so that they increase the potential for nocturnal bronchoconstriction.

To properly evaluate the circadian variation in lung function in asthma, peak flows should be recorded by the patient at specific times throughout the day. Assessments at bedtime, during any awakening period, and in the morning are good indicators of the condition of the airway. Additionally, a peak expiratory flow rate (PEFR) measurement can be made late in the afternoon to determine the time of best lung function. The effectiveness of therapy also can be determined by the PEFR recordings the patient makes at home. Once the patient is stable, there is an objective parameter to follow. A gradual decrease in the PEFR or increase in circadian swings may be an indication of impending problems.

The treatment of nocturnal asthma is based on an understanding of circadian rhythms, pharmacokinetics, and pharmacodynamics. An appropriate approach to the treatment of sleep-related asthma includes intensifying the therapy when the symptoms are at their worst (chronotherapy).

Asthmatics with decreased clearance of secretions due to upper airway disease, sinusitis, or nasal congestion may have poor sleep and nocturnal symptoms. Treatment with oral decongestants, nasal steroid preparations, saline nasal washes, or chest physical therapy may improve symptoms in these asthmatic patients.

The asthmatic patient receiving bronchodilators and steroids also may be experiencing GERD. Reflex bronchoconstriction via the vagal system can occur as the gastric contents irritate the esophageal mucosa. When reflux is an important factor in nocturnal asthma, treatment should include H_2 blockers, bedtime antacids, and elevation of the head of the bed.

Most patients require and benefit from **bronchodilator therapy**. Maximizing dosages to ensure optimal bronchodilatory effects throughout the entire 24-hour day is essential. Long-acting oral and inhaled beta-agonists may be helpful in treating the symptoms of nocturnal asthma, as may long acting theophylline preparations.

The present patient was treated with beta-adrenergic agonists and methylxanthines that were optimized for peak serum levels at 2 to 4 AM.

Clinical Pearls

1. The naturally occurring circadian rhythms play a major role in the pathophysiology of asthma with nocturnal exacerbations.

2. When the circadian pattern variation in pulmonary function approaches 50%, it is an important indicator of potentially severe nighttime symptoms.

3. The prevailing symptoms in sleep-related asthma occur at night, with the peak airflow obstruction occurring between midnight and 6 AM.

REFERENCES

1. Crescioli S, Dal Carobbo A, Maestrelli P. Controlled-release theophylline inhibits early morning airway obstruction and hyperresponsiveness in asthmatic subjects. Ann Allergy Asthma Immunol 1996;77:106–110.
2. Storms WW, Nathan RA, Bodman SF, Byer P. Improving the treatment of nocturnal asthma: Use of an office questionnaire to identify nocturnal asthma symptoms. J Asthma 1996;33:165–168.
3. Van Keimpema AR, Ariaansz M, Raaijmakers JA, et al. Treatment of nocturnal asthma by addition of oral slow-release albuterol to standard treatment in stable asthma patients. J Asthma 1996;33:119–124.
4. Oosterhoff Y, Timens W, Postma DS. The role of airway inflammation in the pathophysiology of nocturnal asthma. Clin Exp Allergy 1995;25:915–921.
5. Chhabra SK. An epidemiological investigation into nocturnal asthma. J Asthma 1995;32:147–150.
6. Martin RJ. Nocturnal asthma. Chest 1995;107:158S–161S.

PATIENT 75

A 46-year-old man with a sore throat and a persistent nonproductive cough

A 46-year-old man presented to his physician's office complaining of persistent cough of 2-week duration. He had tried to alleviate the cough with over-the-counter antitussives, to no avail. Medical history included hypertension which was diagnosed 2 months earlier and for which he had recently started taking captopril.

Physical Examination: Temperature 98.6°; pulse 88; respirations 14; blood pressure 138/92. Chest: clear. Cardiac: normal. Abdomen: normal. Neurologic: alert and oriented, nonfocal.

Laboratory Findings: SpO$_2$ (room air): 96%. Chest radiograph: see below.

Question: What are the most common causes of persistent, chronic cough?

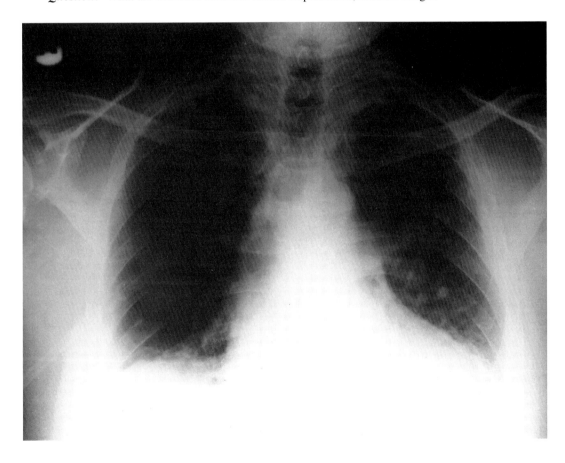

Diagnosis: Captopril-induced cough.

Discussion: Cough can assume great clinical importance, due to both the annoyance of the symptom itself and the potentially serious underlying diseases that may manifest themselves in this way. As a defense mechanism, cough has two main functions: to prevent foreign material from entering the lower respiratory tract and to clear foreign material and excessive secretions from the airway. As a symptom of disease, cough may represent asthma, gastroesophageal reflux, chronic sinusitis, postnasal drip, and a side effect of medication, particularly the angiotensin-converting enzyme (ACE) inhibitors such as captopril. Cough can also be the presenting manifestation of lung cancer, diffuse parenchymal disorders, and mediastinal conditions.

The **mechanics of cough** include three phases. The inspiratory phase consists of a deep and sometimes forceful inspiration through a widely opened glottis. The compressive phase begins with closure of the glottis, continues with active contraction of the expiratory muscles, and ends with sudden opening of the glottis. During expiratory phase, the clearance function of cough is carried out. Intraluminal debris clearance is allowed through coordinated movements of the glottis, respiratory muscles, and tracheobronchial tree.

ACE inhibitor–induced cough is extremely common and is a frequent reason why patients discontinue the drug, either on their own or with a physician's advice. Reports of ACE inhibitor–induced cough range from 5–72% of patients taking the drugs. As cough is often perceived more as an annoyance than as a serious symptom, it is likely that initial study of adverse events related to ACE inhibitors substantially underreported the prevalence of cough in patients taking these medications.

In ACE inhibitor–induced cough, the pathogenesis is thought to be related to an accumulation of inflammatory or proinflammatory mediators (bradykinin, prostaglandins, and/or substance P) in the airway. These mediators increase the sensitivity of the cough reflex. While various bronchodilators and nonsteroidal anti-inflammatory agents have been used to treat ACE inhibitor cough, the recommended treatment is discontinuation of the medication when patients find the cough intolerable. Though the resolution of ACE inhibitor cough may be quick, some patients have reported that their cough persisted for 2 months after stopping the medication.

Recently, a class of antihypertensives that also works on the renin-angiotensin-aldosterone system has been developed. These antihypertensives are antagonists of angiotensin II, and apparently this downstream effect makes the side effect of cough less common.

The present patient's cough disappeared 3 days after discontinuation of the captopril. His hypertension was controlled with atenolol.

Clinical Pearls

1. Healthy people rarely cough persistently. Therefore, the first step in managing patients who complain of chronic cough is to make an accurate diagnosis of its cause.

2. When the chest roentgenogram is normal in a nonsmoker who has not been taking an ACE-inhibitor, the cause of cough is almost always post-nasal drip syndrome, asthma, and/or gastroesophageal reflux disease.

3. Because there is no laboratory test that predicts who will get ACE inhibitor–induced cough, the diagnosis should be considered in any patient who develops cough after initiation of ACE inhibitors.

REFERENCES

1. Fox AJ, Lalloo UG, Belvisi MG, et al. Bradykinin-evoked sensitization of airway sensory nerves: A mechanism for ACE-inhibitor cough. Nat Med 1996;2:814–817.
2. Ludviksdottir D, Bjornsson E, Janson C, et al. Habitual coughing and its association with asthma, anxiety, and gastroesophageal reflux. Chest 1996;109:1262–1268.
3. Mello CJ, Irwin RS, Curley FJ. Predictive values of the character, timing, and complication of chronic cough in diagnosing its cause. Arch Intern Med 1996;156:997–1003.
4. Tomaki M, Ichinose M, Miura M, et al. Angiotensin converting enzyme (ACE) inhibitor-induced cough and substance P. Thorax 1996;51:199–201.
5. Ramsay LE, Yeo WW, ACE inhibitors, angiotensin II antagonists, and cough: The Losartan Cough Study Group. J Hum Hypertens 1995;9(Suppl 5):S51–S54.
6. Wood R. Bronchospasm and cough as adverse reactions to the ACE inhibitors captopril, enalapril, and lisinopril: A controlled retrospective cohort study. Brit J Clin Pharm 1995;39:265–270.
7. Yeo WW, Chadwick IG, Kraskiewicz M, et al. Resolution of ACE inhibitor cough: Changes in subjective cough and responses to inhaled capsaicin, intradermal bradykinin and substance-P. Brit J Clin Pharm 1995;40:423–429.

INDEX

Page numbers in **bold face** indicate complete cases.

Endotracheal tubes
  kinks in, 151, 152
  malposition of, **175–176**
  mucus plug obstruction of, 151, 152
End-tidal pressure of carbon dioxide (PET_{CO_2}), in
    mechanical ventilation monitoring, 176
Eosinophilia, Wegener's granulomatosis-related, 118
Epigastric pain, hepatitis B-related, 127
Epiglottitis, acute, **125–126**
L-Epinephrine, as laryngeal edema treatment, 34, 35
Epistaxis, nasopharyngeal carcinoma-related, 96
Epstein-Barr virus, as nasopharyngeal carcinoma cause, 97
Erythema nodosum, 43
Escherichia coli, as meningitis cause, 131
Esophago-gastrectomy, as pneumothorax cause, **150–152**
Ethambutol, use as tuberculosis treatment, 174
Exercise, therapeutic, by cystic fibrosis patients, 166
Exercise testing, for exercise-induced bronchospasm
    detection, 111
Expiratory airflow obstruction, chronic obstructive
    pulmonary disease-related, 6
Extracorporeal membrane oxygenation (ECMO)
  as adult and infant respiratory distress syndrome treat-
    ment, 71
  as congenital diaphragmatic hernia treatment, 73
Extubation
  as subglottic edema cause, **33–35**
  as tracheal injury cause, 53

Face, burn injury to, 63, **138–139**
Facial anatomy, use in airway assessment, 184
Factor V Leiden deficiency, 40
Fatigue
  bronchiectasis-related, 18
  chronic obstructive pulmonary disease-related, 6
  hepatitis B-related, 127, 128
  lung cancer-related, 119
  toxic ingestion-related, 21, 22
FEV_1/FVC (forced expiratory volume in one second/forced
    vital capacity) ratio, normal versus abnormal, 111
Fever
  acute chest syndrome-related, 26
  cystic fibrosis-related, 162
  empyema-related, 3
  epiglottitis-related, 125, 126
  heat stroke-related, 136, 137
  laryngotracheobronchitis-related, 112, 113
  meningitis-related, 130, 131
  pneumonia-related, 170, 186
  sickle cell anemia-related, 25
  tuberculosis-related, 173, 174
Fibrosis, pulmonary
  idiopathic, 108
  interstitial, 108
  mediastinal, histoplasmosis-related, 99, 100
  oxygen therapy-related, **107–109**
  silicosis-related, 134
  systemic lupus erythematosus-related, 91
"Fighting the ventilator," **153–155**
FiO_2 (fractional concentration of carbon dioxide in inspired
    gas), of low-flow oxygen therapy systems, 178, 179
Fistula
  bronchopleural, **50–51**
  tracheo-inominate, 157
Flail chest, with pulmonary contusion, **147–149**
Fluid replacement therapy, for heat stroke, 137
Flumazil, use as benzodiazepine antagonist, 58
Flutter device, 166
Forced expiratory volume in one second/forced vital
    capacity ratio, 111

Foreign bodies, aspiration of, 30
Fractional concentration of carbon dioxide in inspired gas
    (FiO_2), of low-flow oxygen therapy systems, 178, 179
Fractures
  hypovolemic shock associated with, **87–89**
  thoracic, as flail chest cause, **147–149**
Functional residual capacity (FRC), in amyotrophic lateral
    sclerosis, 66

Gag reflex, 34, 46
Gallium scan, for sarcoidosis diagnosis, 43, 44
Gamma-aminobutyric acid, interaction with
    benzodiazepines, 58
Gastric contents, aspiration of
  by head injury patients, 46
  as lung abscess cause, 187
Gastric lavage, orogastric tube placement in, 22
Gastroesophageal reflux, 189, 192
Granuloma
  eosinophilic, 123
  histoplasmosis-related, 99
  sarcoidosis-related, 43, 44

Haemophilus influenzae infections
  in alcoholic patients, 187
  epiglottitis as, 113, 126
  meningitis as, 131
  pneumonia as, **23–24**
  in sickle cell disease patients, 26
  in systemic lupus erythematosus patients, 91
Headache
  intracerebral hemorrhage-related, 45
  meningitis-related, 130, 131
  persistent, 36
Head and neck cancer, 97
Head and neck injury, **15–17**
  flail chest associated with, 148
  as nosocomial pneumonia risk factor, **45–47**
Healthcare workers, hepatitis exposure risk of, 128,
    129
Heart murmur, patent ductus arteriosis-related, 49
Heat inhalation injury, of upper airway, 63, **138–139**
Heat stroke, **136–137**
Heliox, 34
Hemithorax, opacified, 30
Hemoptysis
  bronchiectasis-related, 20
  lung cancer-related, 29, 30
  Wegener's granulomatosis-related, 117, 118
Hemorrhage
  alveolar, 91, 92
  hypertensive intracerebral, **45–47**
  as hypovolemic shock cause, 88
Hemothorax, flail chest-related, 148
Hepatic failure, fulminant, 128, 129
Hepatitis, isoniazid-related, 174
Hepatitis A, 128, 129
Hepatitis B, acute viral, **127–129**
Hepatitis C, 128
Hepatorenal syndrome, 128
Hernia, congenital diaphragmatic, **72–74**
Histoplasmosis, **98–100**, 187
  AIDS-related, 10, 99, 100
Human immunodeficiency virus (HIV) infection, as
    tuberculosis risk factor, 174
Hyaline membrane, oxygen therapy-related formation of,
    109
Hyaline membrane disease. *See* Infant respiratory distress
    syndrome
Hydrogen chloride, as chemical burn cause, 63